Workbook for

Elsevier's Veterinary Assisting Textbook

Workbook for

Elsevier's Veterinary Assisting Textbook

Fourth Edition

Ann Wortinger, BIS, LVT, VTS (ECC) (SAIM) (Nutrition), Elite FFCP
Lecturer, Content Development Coordinator
Appalachian State University
Boone, North Carolina

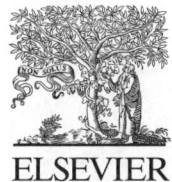

ELSEVIER

Elsevier
3251 Riverport Lane
St. Louis, Missouri 63043

WORKBOOK FOR ELSEVIER'S VETERINARY ASSISTING
TEXTBOOK, FOURTH EDITION

ISBN: 978-0-443-11714-5

Notice

Practitioners and researchers must always rely on their own experience and knowledge in evaluating and using any information, methods, compounds or experiments described herein. Because of rapid advances in the medical sciences, in particular, independent verification of diagnoses and drug dosages should be made. To the fullest extent of the law, no responsibility is assumed by Elsevier, authors, editors or contributors for any injury and/or damage to persons or property as a matter of products liability, negligence or otherwise, or from any use or operation of any methods, products, instructions, or ideas contained in the material herein.

Previous editions copyrighted 2021, 2017 and 2013.

Content Strategist: Melissa Rawe, Samantha Hart
Content Development Manager: Danielle Frazier
Senior Content Development Specialist: Maria Broeker
Publishing Services Manager: Deepthi Unni
Senior Project Manager: Beula Christopher

Printed in United States of America

Last digit is the print number: 9   8   7   6   5   4   3   2   1

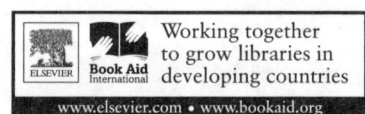

Coming on board for the fourth edition has been a labor of love for my dear friend Dr. Margi Sirois, who was responsible for the previous editions. She is loved and missed, and I enjoyed the opportunity to hear her voice again as I progressed through this edition.

My husband, Todd for all the support and for kindly leaving me alone in the office so that I could get all the work done! He, unfortunately, also gets to be the recipient of all of my frustrations and questions at the end of the day.

My feline editorial staff consists of Dusty, our blind Detroit stray, whose position was as chief lap warmer and contributor, Poppy, our TNR rescue, has stepped up to be my Zoom buddy and research assistant. Jack, Millie, and BeeGee have the enviable job of seeing how much hair can be released on my desk, as well as making much use of the window cat-ledge in my office. All of the cats had the unfailing ability to know exactly which book or article I was currently working out of or would need next. You very kindly marked it with your furry bodies. Supervision was conducted from my lap, my desk, and the pet stairs. How does anyone work without a feline editorial staff?

Preface

Veterinary assistants play a vital role in the veterinary health care team. An educated assistant working directly with a credentialed veterinary technician can help create a powerful team that greatly improves the ability of the veterinarian to attend to animals in their care. Veterinary assistants are also involved in many of the business aspects of veterinary practice and often work closely with management staff in the practice. This book was designed to aid the veterinary assistant in obtaining the knowledge and skills required to assist the veterinary technician and veterinarian in the care of animals, as well as skills needed to contribute to the smooth functioning of the business side of a companion animal veterinary practice.

Veterinary assistants are most effective when they have a strong understanding of the flow of work in the practice and the roles of each of the members of the veterinary health care team. This information is contained in each chapter. Each chapter begins with learning objectives, a chapter outline, and keywords. "Critical Concepts" throughout each chapter highlight important points and provide helpful tips to improve knowledge and skills. Recommended readings provide additional sources of detailed information on the topics. Step-by-step procedures are included for all commonly performed skills expected of veterinary assistants. Ample illustrations are included, and tables are used to provide a summary and handy reference for vital information.

The majority of the material for the text is derived from published material in several other textbooks, including *Principles and Practice of Veterinary Technology*, fifth edition; *Front Office Management for the Veterinary Team*, third edition; *Laboratory Procedures for Veterinary Technicians*, Seventh edition; *Animal Restraint for Veterinary Professionals*, third edition; *McCurnin's Clinical Textbook for Veterinary Technicians*, 10th edition; *Diagnostic Parasitology for Veterinary Technicians*, Sixth edition; and *Clinical Anatomy and Physiology for Veterinary Technicians*, fourth edition.

The text is designed to adhere to the model curricula for veterinary assistant training as published by the Association of Veterinary Technician Educators and the National Association of Veterinary Technicians in America. Additional information regarding farm animals, exotic animals, and alternate diagnostic imaging techniques is also included for those programs that cover expanded topics. New to this edition is the chapter *Hospice, Grief, and Pet Loss*. It discusses the human-animal bond and stages of grief as well as other principles that prepare students for the veterinary assistant's role in helping an owner through pet loss. Programs for the training of veterinary assistants will find this a valuable resource for providing details on tasks performed by veterinary assistants as well as the roles of all the members of the veterinary health care team.

WORKBOOK

The accompanying workbook includes definitions of key terms, review questions, case presentations, clinical applications, illustration labeling and identification, photo-based quizzes, matching questions, completion questions (fill-in-the-blank type), and multiple-choice questions. Each chapter in the workbook corresponds to a chapter in the textbook and reinforces the essential information of the chapter through the use of various exercises and test questions. Students are encouraged to read and review the chapter before attempting to work through the related exercises in the workbook. Chapter objectives provided in the textbook are reiterated in the workbook to help students focus on the material and concepts that they are expected to learn and understand how this is to be applied in the veterinary clinic setting.

EVOLVE RESOURCES

Assets for Instructors

Instructors can activate the complete teaching experience that comes with this book by registering at http://evolve.elsevier.com/Elsevier/vetassisting/. Resources include TEACH, a popular and useful resource providing one-stop classroom planning with lectures, activities, and more. Register today and also gain access to the electronic image collection, test bank, PowerPoint lecture outlines, workbook answer key, and Chapter Pretests.

Assets for Students

Practice quizzes for students are brand-new with this edition. This resource is included with a print or eBook purchase and can be activated by redeeming the code on the inside front cover. Over 200 multiple-choice questions are separated into chapter assessments and provide the opportunity for students to actively recall information presented in each chapter.

Acknowledgments

This book would not have been possible without the hard work of the many authors and contributors to the previously published textbooks from which much of this volume is derived, especially that of Dr. Margi Sirois, who was responsible for all of the previous editions of this book. I thank them all for their efforts.

**Ann Wortinger, BIS, LVT, VTS (ECC) (SAIM)
(NUTRITION), Elite FFCP**

Contents

Workbook for

Elsevier's Veterinary Assisting Textbook

1 Overview of the Veterinary Profession

LEARNING OBJECTIVES

After reviewing this chapter, the reader will be able to:

- Describe the educational requirements of veterinary team members.
- Define appropriate nomenclature describing veterinary personnel.
- Identify the duties of the members of the veterinary health care team.
- Recognize professional organizations supporting veterinary medicine.
- Discuss ethical issues and guidelines relevant to the veterinary profession.
- List and describe general categories of laws relevant to the veterinary profession.
- Define laws protecting veterinary employees against physical injury, sexual harassment, and discrimination.
- Explain laws relating to ensuring quality veterinary service.

LISTS

1. List seven possible members of the veterinary team:
   1. _____
   2. _____
   3. _____
   4. _____
   5. _____
   6. _____
   7. _____

2. List nine responsibilities of a veterinary assistant:
   1. _____
   2. _____
   3. _____
   4. _____
   5. _____
   6. _____
   7. _____
   8. _____
   9. _____

3. List seven areas or zones in a veterinary practice:
   1. _____
   2. _____
   3. _____
   4. _____
   5. _____
   6. _____
   7. _____

4. List three key safety steps for operating machinery and moving parts of equipment:
   1. _____
   2. _____
   3. _____

5. List the laws that ensure the quality of veterinary services:
   1. _____
   2. _____

6. List the laws that provide a safe business environment:
   1. _____
   2. _____
   3. _____

7. List the seven areas of safety in the workplace that OSHA addresses:
   1. _____
   2. _____
   3. _____
   4. _____
   5. _____
   6. _____
   7. _____

8. List the two hazards to be concerned about during bathing and dipping procedures:
   1. _____
   2. _____

9. List the five zoonotic hazards encountered in veterinary practice:
   1. _____
   2. _____
   3. _____
   4. _____
   5. _____

10. List the steps for radiation safety:
    1. _____
    2. _____
    3. _____
    4. _____
    5. _____

11. List the types of veterinary practices:
    1. _____
    2. _____
    3. _____
    4. _____
    5. _____

MATCHING

Match the group with its purpose.

1. _____ Academy
2. _____ NAVTA
3. _____ Society

A. Fosters high standards of veterinary care and promotes the veterinary health care team
B. Association of professionals with common interests
C. Specialty group involved in credentialing of individuals

Match the team member with the description.

1. _____ Veterinary Assistant
2. _____ Veterinary Technician
3. _____ Veterinary Technologist
4. _____ Veterinary Technician Specialist
5. _____ Veterinarian

A. A person who has graduated from a 2-year AVMA-accredited program
B. A person who has graduated from a 4-year CVTEA-accredited program
C. A person with the training of a clinical aide
D. A person who has graduated from a 4-year AVMA-accredited program receiving a Doctor of Veterinary Medicine degree
E. Credentialed technician who meets requirements established by an academy

MULTIPLE CHOICE

1. A person fired because of their sex or race is protected under which federal law?
   a. EEO
   b. FDA
   c. SSD
   d. PPE

2. Which federal agency is responsible for combating the abuse of controlled substances?
   a. DEA
   b. USDA
   c. NFLA
   d. FDA

3. How can exposure to formalin be minimized?
   a. Wear latex gloves when pouring from the larger storage container into the small transport containers
   b. Dumping any unused liquid down the drain
   c. Using premeasured vials for transport
   d. Only mixing up the amount of powder needed daily with a predetermined volume of distilled water

4. Under what circumstances should extension electrical cords be used?
   a. When there are not enough electrical outlets for all the equipment needed
   b. When it is anticipated that the floors may become wet
   c. For temporary use
   d. In high-traffic areas

5. The veterinary team consists of which individuals?
   a. The veterinarian, veterinary technician, assistants, receptionists, and hospital managers
   b. Stockholders, clients, and local businesses
   c. Animal control officers, veterinarians, and kennel staff
   d. Rescues, TNR groups, and shelters

6. Who is responsible for using a veterinary assistant appropriately and ethically?
   a. Veterinarian
   b. CSR
   c. Veterinary technician
   d. Client

7. Which organization provides free membership with access to affordable online continuing education?
   a. USDA
   b. VSPN
   c. VHMA
   d. OSHA

8. A society can include which members of the veterinary team?
   a. Any interested member
   b. Credentialed veterinary technicians
   c. Certified practice manager
   d. Licensed veterinarians

9. Which member of the veterinary team does not require credentialing?
   a. Veterinarian
   b. Veterinary technician
   c. Veterinary assistant
   d. Veterinary technologist

10. What are duties that can be delegated to an assistant?
    a. Surgery
    b. Writing prescriptions
    c. Diagnosis of common problems
    d. Laboratory testing

11. What activity can result in increased productivity from the veterinarian?
    a. Coming in 2 hours before the staff
    b. Shortening their surgical time
    c. Delegating tasks
    d. Getting more CE

12. Which team member can prescribe medications?
    a. Veterinarian
    b. Veterinary technician
    c. Veterinary assistant
    d. Practice manager

13. Credentialed veterinary technicians have attended what type of school?
    a. Community college
    b. AVMA-approved program
    c. Private colleges
    d. Community vocational schools

14. What condition in the waiting room can contribute to increased stress for clients and their pets?
    a. Pheromone diffusers
    b. Being acknowledged by the CSR as soon as they arrive
    c. Being directed to a specific dog or cat area
    d. Overcrowding

15. What type of veterinary practice treats dogs, cats, horses, cattle, and sheep?
    a. Companion animal
    b. Livestock
    c. Exotics
    d. Mixed

16. Veterinarians who have special expertise in one aspect of medicine can often be found in what type of practices?
    a. Mixed
    b. Companion
    c. Referral
    d. Exotic

17. What are typical items found in the retail area of a veterinary clinic?
    a. Surgical instruments
    b. Foods and leashes
    c. Antibiotics
    d. Heartworm test kits

18. Where is the general practice layout of the diagnostic areas of treatment, radiology, and surgery located?
    a. In the back of the practice
    b. Closest to the waiting room
    c. Next to the examination room
    d. Immediately behind the reception desk

19. Chronically underfeeding but not starving an animal is an example of what kind of problem?
    a. Ethical
    b. Legal
    c. Ignoring the human-animal bond
    d. Animal baiting

20. Which laws govern how a veterinarian, veterinary technician, and veterinary assistant can perform their duties?
    a. Federal
    b. State
    c. County
    d. City

21. What term is used to describe a special, healthy relationship between people and their pets?
    a. Human-animal bond
    b. Common law bond
    c. Codependent bond
    d. Enabling bond

22. When handling a scared or defensive animal, what piece of equipment can be safely used to prevent injury to them and yourself?
    a. Squeeze chute
    b. Big, fluffy towel
    c. 1–2 extra sets of hands to hold them down
    d. There is no safe way to handle these animals, and care should be denied

23. What is the purpose of a dosimetry badge?
    a. To measure scatter radiation received during x-rays
    b. To provide additional identification to the staff
    c. To monitor the exposure of staff to halogenated gasses
    d. To monitor exposure to ultraviolet radiation

24. Under what conditions does the National Fire Protection Association recommend that you do NOT attempt to fight a fire?
    a. A fire extinguisher is nearby
    b. The location is confined and localized
    c. The fire could block your exit
    d. You had training on how to use the extinguisher last week

25. If an action by a veterinarian causes injury to a patient through negligence, under what law can the owners sue the veterinarian?
    a. The State Practice Act
    b. The FDA Legal Claims Act
    c. Common law malpractice
    d. The College of Veterinary Medicine

26. Needles and syringes are typically disposed of in red waste containers. Why are they not disposed of in the regular trash?
    a. They are medical waste
    b. Items in the red container can be reused
    c. They can be recycled
    d. It can help to decrease the cost of disposal

27. Which term refers to a defined system of moral principles that determines appropriate behavior and actions within a specific group?
    a. Common laws
    b. Practice distractors
    c. Ethics
    d. Human-animal bond

28. According to OSHA, who is responsible for ensuring that the workplace is free from recognized hazards?
    a. The employee
    b. The veterinarians
    c. The employer
    d. The police department

29. Why is the one-handed needle recapping technique recommended?
    a. To help prevent needlestick injuries
    b. To ensure manual dexterity
    c. To keep the needles sharp for reuse
    d. To allow the syringes to be easily disconnected from the needle

30. A Hazardous Materials Plan is a strategic component of which law?
    a. The Practice Safety Law
    b. The Controlled Substance Act
    c. Right to Know Law
    d. Common law

31. When would wearing personal hearing protection be appropriate?
    a. Shoveling snow off the front walk
    b. End-of-shift disinfection of examination and treatment rooms
    c. Caring for an animal in the isolation ward
    d. Cleaning the dog kennels

32. What PPE is NOT worn when taking radiographs?
    a. Lead gown
    b. Leather gloves
    c. Dosimetry badge
    d. Thyroid shield

33. What does a dosimetry badge measure?
    a. Sterilization of surgical packs
    b. Disinfection procedure effectiveness
    c. Scatter radiation
    d. Vaccination status

34. A veterinary technologist has graduated from what type of AVMA-accredited program?
    a. 1-year
    b. 2-year
    c. 3-year
    d. 4-year

35. Negligence that causes injury to the patient is legally called what?
    a. Malpractice
    b. Standard of care
    c. An OSHA violation
    d. Freedom of speech

36. A veterinary technician has graduated from what type of AVMA-accredited program?
    a. 1-year
    b. 2-year
    c. 3-year
    d. 4-year

37. Which legal act is designed to provide a safe workplace for everyone working in any business affecting commerce?
    a. OSHA
    b. DEA
    c. SDS
    d. FSLA

38. When performing a medicated bath, what PPE would you be expected to wear?
    a. Lead apron, thyroid shield, and lead gloves
    b. Gloves, masks, and goggles
    c. Lab coat, sturdy shoes, and a watch with a second hand
    d. Athletic shoes, blue jeans, and a ball cap

39. What is defined as a special, healthy relationship between people and their pets?
    a. Codependency
    b. Puppy mills
    c. ASPCA
    d. Human-animal bond

40. A Hazardous Materials Plan uses what type of information on chemicals found in the hospital?
    a. SDS sheets
    b. OSHA plans
    c. EEO handouts
    d. Controlled substance classifications

41. When a veterinary technician has graduated from an AVMA-accredited program, passed the VTNE, and maintains certification, registration, or licensure in the state in which they live, they are said to be what?
    a. Covered
    b. Credentialed
    c. Accredited
    d. Practicing

42. Which persons in the hospital have the training of a clinical aide; excel at physical restraint, basic laboratory skills, patient care, and client relations; and can assist veterinary technicians and veterinarians?
    a. Veterinary assistant
    b. Veterinary technician
    c. Veterinarian
    d. Client service representative

43. What type of veterinary practice specializes in treating family pets?
    a. Mixed animal
    b. Large animal
    c. Companion animal
    d. Multipurpose

44. What is defined by the failure to exercise the necessary legal obligation of skill and diligence in treating a patient?
    a. Negligence
    b. Valid V-C-P relationship
    c. OSHA violation
    d. Overdose

45. A state practice act defines what limitations?
    a. What a veterinary assistant can do
    b. The practice of veterinary medicine and surgery
    c. What clients a hospital can see
    d. The standard of dress

46. The requirement for a list of chemicals found in a hospital is part of what law?
    a. Controlled Substance Act
    b. Ionizing Radiation Control Act
    c. Distraction Avoidance Law
    d. The Right to Know Law

CASE SCENARIO

In your state, the practice defines skills only performed by a veterinarian as diagnose, prognose, prescribe, and do surgery. Skills performed by a credentialed veterinary technician are defined as place an intravenous catheter and perform venipuncture, administer vaccines, induce and maintain anesthesia, intubate, and perform surgical wound closure. Skills performed by a veterinary assistant are not defined in the Practice Act; however, all of the above skills are not allowed by anyone other than those persons designated.

Let us follow Harvey on his first visit to All Friends Animal Hospital. You will provide who can perform the highlighted skills as we move through Harvey's visit.

Harvey's new owner, Cindy, has called All Friends to book an appointment for an initial evaluation with a possible neuter. Harvey is a 15-month-old mixed-breed male dog that Cindy has recently adopted after a close family friend passed away.

1. **Who answers the call and books the appointment?**
   _____
   _____
   _____

2. **Why?**
   _____
   _____
   _____

Harvey is scheduled to avoid in a fasted state in case surgery is an option for him. Cindy calls from the parking lot to let you know that they have arrived. It had previously been explained to Cindy that the hospital policy was to have Harvey move directly from the parking lot into the examination room with a brief stop at the scales. This process helps to keep Harvey's fear, anxiety, and stress lower during his visit.

3. **Who brings Harvey into the examination room and why?**
   _____
   _____

Harvey weighs 86# on the walk-on scale. On physical examination, he is bright, alert, and responsive, with normal temperature, pulse, and respirations. Cindy is asked what type of food he is eating, if there are any other animals in the house, and if she has any concerns. On the previous owner's records, it is evident that he is not currently on vaccines and has not been on heartworm preventative nor has he been tested for heartworm disease this year.

4. **Who can conduct the physical examination and collect the history?**
   _____
   _____

Hospital policy is that all dogs having surgery must have negative heartworm and fecal tests and can be vaccinated on the day of surgery. Cindy elects to have the heartworm test done, picks up 12 months of preventative, and wants to bring him up-to-date on his vaccines. Blood needs to be collected for a 4Dx Snap test from IDEXX (this tests for heartworm, Lyme disease, *Ehrlichia*, and *Anaplasma*, all diseases found in this area) and for a presurgical chemistry panel and CBC. Core vaccines in this area are distemper/parvovirus combo, flu, and 3-year rabies.

5. **Who can collect the blood?**
   _____
   _____
   _____

6. **Who can run the 4Dx, fecal, chemistry, and CBC tests?**
   _____
   _____
   _____

7. **Who can give the vaccines?**
   _____
   _____
   _____

Harvey's presurgical blood work is within normal range, and his 4Dx is negative for all diseases. He is cleared for his surgery today. Based on his weight, his preanesthetic, anesthetic, and postoperative pain drugs are drawn up, and the surgical suite is set up for a neuter. At the assigned time, the anesthetic drugs this doctor prefers are administered, Harvey is intubated and started on anesthesia. His surgical site is clipped of hair, and an initial surgical scrub is done outside the surgical suite.

8. Who can draw up the preanesthetic, anesthetic, and postoperative pain drugs?

_____

_____

_____

9. Who can administer the preanesthetic drugs?

_____

_____

_____

10. Who can administer the anesthetic drugs and intubate Harvey?

_____

_____

_____

11. Who can do the surgical clip and scrub?

_____

_____

_____

Harvey is moved to the surgical suite, where he is positioned on the table, and a final scrub applied. The surgical pack, surgical gown, gloves, suture material, and scalpel blade are all opened. The doctor performs their presurgical scrub, dons their surgical gown and gloves, and is tied into their gown. For this surgery the technician will be assisting, as Harvey is a bigger dog.

12. Who performs the final scrub and positions Harvey on the table?

_____

_____

_____

13. Who opens all the packs and materials?

_____

_____

_____

14. Who ties the doctor and technician into their gowns?

_____

_____

_____

The surgical incision is made, and the testicles are ligated and removed. The muscle and skin layers are closed. The postoperative pain medications are given, and Harvey is recovered from the anesthetic.

15. Who performs the surgical incision and surgery?

_____

_____

_____

16. Who performs the skin closure?

_____

_____

_____

17. Who administers the postoperative drugs?

_____

_____

_____

18. Who recovers and extubates Harvey?

_____

_____

_____

Harvey's recovery goes well, and he is scheduled to go home that evening. While he is recovering, the discharge instructions are completed following the routine hospital template. He will receive 5 days of pain medicines that will be sent home for Cindy to administer. He will also be sent home with a yearly supply of heartworm and flea and tick preventatives. Harvey has no external sutures, so a suture removal will not be necessary. Cindy comes back at 4:30 p.m. to pick him up. She pays her bill before Harvey is brought up.

19. Who collects the money for the bill?

_____

_____

_____

20. Who goes through the discharge instructions and explains about the pain and heartworm medications?

_____

_____

_____

2 Office Procedures and Client Relations

LEARNING OBJECTIVES

After reviewing this chapter, the reader will be able to:

- Describe the importance of informed consent.
- Clarify admitting and discharge instructions.
- Identify effective and professional discharge sheets.
- Define and educate clients regarding pet health insurance.
- Identify a completed medical record.
- Identify and use problem-oriented medical record and subjective, objective, assessment, and plan record formats.
- Identify methods used to accurately and efficiently maintain inventory.
- Develop effective phone techniques.
- Identify techniques for handling multiple phone lines.
- Describe methods to greet clients effectively.
- Differentiate forms used in the veterinary practice.

FILL IN THE BLANK

1. Teamwork helps facilitate _____ for clients and employees.

2. The quality of voice is a combination of _____, _____, _____, and _____.

3. The ultimate goal of inventory costs is that they should total _____% to _____% of the overall income of the practice.

4. To put _____ at ease, a warm welcome from and accessibility of team members are must.

5. The client's experience starts with the first _____ and ends when the practice has _____ up after the visit.

6. If the client has to call the practice to receive test results, this can leave a _____ impression.

7. The receptionist should answer the phone within _____ rings.

8. Information can be misinterpreted, especially over the phone; a pet's condition must never be _____ over the phone!

9. Appointment schedules should be developed to _____ production while _____ client wait time.

10. _____ _____ are issued by the US Department of Agriculture and by the state and may be required for interstate and international travel.

11. A valid _____ relationship must exist for a veterinarian to dispense prescription products.

12. When the receptionist details the entire _____ for the client, it shows the total charges for the visit.

13. A collections agency's report can remain on a client's credit report for _____ years.

14. On release from the hospital, patients must be released with _____ instructions.

15. Indemnity insurance offers _____ for treatment of injured and sick pets.

16. A _____ is defined as the amount an owner pays monthly or annually to maintain an insurance policy for a pet.

17. A _____ is the amount an owner must pay before the insurance company will offer compensation.

18. A copay is the _____ that the owner is responsible for after the deductible has been met.

19. Insurance may be denied because of a _____ condition—an abnormality transmitted by genes from parent to offspring.

20. Backing up documents _____ prevents thieves from stealing the most current copy of data from the practice if they are removing all the computer equipment or if a fire or natural disaster occurs.

21. Costs associated with expired medications, ordering, shipping, insurance, and taxes are _____ costs.

22. Surgical patients must be examined within _____ hours prior to receiving anesthesia.

23. Small animals flying in the United States may require an _____.

24. A medical record is a legal document that must be maintained for _____ years if the client has not returned to the practice.

25. The most common error made is not documenting the communication with the owner regarding the _____ of the patient.

26. _____ is the goal number of inventory turns each practice should have each year.

27. When a current client-patient-veterinarian relationship exists, a _____ product can be sold.

28. _____ is one of the largest expenses in the practice.

29. Practices may add a _____ fee as well as a minimum prescription charge.

30. Clients draw preliminary conclusions within the first _____ to _____ minutes of entering the building.

SHORT ANSWER

1. Explain why an orthopedic appointment is given more time than a yearly vaccination appointment.

2. Describe how a lack of eye contact can create a negative impression for the client.

3. How do reminder calls help the practice and the clients?

4. How can dropping a pet off at the clinic be of great service to the client?

5. How can you greet a client if you are on the phone or already helping another client?

6. Explain why most new patient/client forms have to include a phone number and driver's license number.

7. Explain what a blanket consent form is and why it is not the best form to use.

8. If a clinic uses paperless medical records, why is it important that all documentation be done in a timely manner?

9. What are SOPs, and why are they so useful in the veterinary practice?

_____
_____
_____
_____
_____
_____
_____
_____

10. Give three examples of products that can be sold by a veterinarian only when the relationship exists between the client and patient.

_____
_____
_____
_____
_____
_____
_____

MULTIPLE CHOICE

1. The stock level that an item reaches before it is reordered is referred to as what?
   a. Expiration date
   b. Reorder point
   c. Inventory level
   d. Sale date

2. How is shrinkage defined?
   a. A contraction in supply due to market demands
   b. A decision to have less product on hand
   c. When a product is unavailable due to backorders
   d. Loss of product without explanation

3. Informed consent forms can be signed under what conditions?
   a. All information regarding the procedure has been provided
   b. When surgical procedures are scheduled, and the risks are clearly defined
   c. Health certificates between states are needed for air travel
   d. To attest proof of rabies vaccination in the event of euthanasia

4. Which person is responsible for signing a rabies certificate?
   a. The person who administers the vaccine
   b. The CSR who fills in the client and patient information
   c. The supervising technician
   d. The veterinarian

5. The increased use of what can contribute to decreased euthanasia rates for individual patients?
   a. Insurance
   b. Vaccines
   c. Premium food
   d. Retractable leashes

6. What information needs to be recorded in the record when speaking with a client on the phone or through email and text?
   a. The time and date of the communication
   b. Any recommendations or changes in care
   c. What form of contact occurred
   d. The date of the last visit to establish they have been in within the previous 6 months

7. When is payment collected for services for any animal admitted to the hospital?
   a. Before the discharge
   b. After the discharge
   c. Within 7 days if using credit
   d. Within 14 days if using cash

8. How much should a product markup be for the practice to break even?
   a. 10%
   b. 20%
   c. 30%
   d. 40%

9. What information is important for new puppy or kitten owners to receive after their first visit?
   a. The anticipated adult size for the animal
   b. Legal statutes for that area
   c. Parasite and vaccine schedules
   d. The best place to purchase toys and food

10. What must have occurred for a prescription product to be dispensed?
    a. The veterinarian must have a valid relationship with the client and the patient
    b. The client has visited the clinic within the past year
    c. Proof of vaccinations has been received
    d. The signs described by the client must be clear and concise

11. For a new patient, whether they have been spayed or neutered is provided under what part of the form?
    a. Vitals
    b. Presenting complaint
    c. Body condition
    d. History

12. How often does a physical inventory need to be done when using a computer system to track hospital inventory?
    a. Monthly
    b. Every 6 months
    c. Every 12 months
    d. This no longer needs to be done

13. A vaccine certificate needs to include what information?
    a. Site the vaccine was given in
    b. When the next vaccine is due
    c. The manufacturer and expiration date
    d. The date of graduation for the veterinarian

14. What is the most used medical record format?
    a. SOAP
    b. POMR
    c. AAHA
    d. SOP

15. Medical records, both electronic and hard copy, are the legal property of who?
    a. The client
    b. The state
    c. The practice
    d. The veterinarian

16. How is patient information entered on the master problem list?
    a. Alphabetically
    b. In order of severity
    c. Client level of concern
    d. Chronologically

17. How are the instructions for medication and rechecks provided after a procedure has been performed?
    a. Verbally
    b. Written handout
    c. Following a standard on your website
    d. The client has been here before, these instructions are not needed

18. For medications needed by an animal, but not stocked at the hospital, what options are available?
    a. Call it in to a human pharmacy
    b. Order from your distributor and ask the client to wait
    c. Send home another medication, but do not tell the client
    d. Only veterinary-approved medications can be given to animals; another drug will have to be chosen

19. The veterinarian has recommended that a client pick up a medication at their local pharmacy that does not require a prescription. What type of product is this?
    a. Controlled
    b. Restricted
    c. Free-choice
    d. OTC

20. Health certificates are issued by the state and what federal agency?
    a. USDA
    b. FDA
    c. OSHA
    d. AVMA

21. When an animal is admitted to the hospital for a surgical procedure, what type of consent form is most often used?
    a. Blanket
    b. Financial
    c. Anesthesia
    d. Euthanasia

22. Where are subjective observations, objective findings, assessment, and plan found?
    a. Patient history
    b. POMR form
    c. Hospital website
    d. State Practice Act

23. What is the percentage of charges for which the owner is responsible after the deductible has been met called?
    a. Copay
    b. Deductible
    c. Premium
    d. Coinsurance

24. The amount an owner must pay before the insurance company will offer compensation is called what?
    a. Copay
    b. Deductible
    c. Premium
    d. Coinsurance

25. What term describes the loss of product without explanation?
    a. Shrinkage
    b. Contraction
    c. Expiration
    d. Wastage

26. A defensive body posture is seen in what forms?
    a. Leaning in
    b. Slumped over
    c. Arms crossed
    d. Hands in scrub pockets

27. What disease is *not* covered for in a DA2LPP vaccine?
    a. Adenovirus type 2
    b. Pox virus
    c. Parvovirus

28. On the SOAP, when listing diseases the patient could have, this is called what?
    a. Rule-outs
    b. Scratch-outs
    c. Rule-ins
    d. All ins

29. What information is required on a prescription label?
    a. The client's name, address, and phone number
    b. The patient's age, sex, and breed
    c. The veterinarian's name, address, and home phone number
    d. The name of the drug, strength, and expiration date

30. If a medication is to be given twice daily, how is this written on the prescription label?
    a. Give every 12 hours
    b. PO SID
    c. Give TID
    d. Give as directed

CASE SCENARIO

Ms. Kulwicki has brought in her newly adopted dog, Jenny, for a wellness visit, vaccines, and preventative. She got her at **the local adoption event sponsored by the Humane Society**.

While Jenny is **14 months old, already spayed, and up to date on her vaccines**, Ms. Kulwicki would like to transfer Jenny's care to your clinic and ensure she is ready for her new life.

On her initial examination, **her weight was 45#**, and her **body condition score was 3/5. T—101.5°F, HR—85 bpm, RR—20 bpm**. She is being fed **Purina ONE dry food, 2 c. twice daily, with fresh baby carrots for treats**. Her last vaccines were 1 month ago, and she **completed her DA2LPP series** and **initial rabies** vaccine. Ms. Kulwicki brought the vaccine schedule provided by the Humane Society.

Dr. Guthery wants to **vaccinate Jenny for flu,** *Bordetella***, and Lyme disease**. Before the vaccines, a **4D × test** is done to ensure she does not have heartworm disease, *Ehrlichia*, *Anaplasma*, or Lyme disease. All of these tests are negative. Jenny is sent home with a **12-month supply of Simparica Trio**, as she is an avid hiker, and Ms. Kulwicki wants to make sure that Jenny can go into the woods with her safely. **Jenny will get one pill by mouth once monthly**.

You explain that Dr. Guthery feels that Jenny is at her full adult size and weight, and further weight gain would be undesired. She does have a **mild ear infection in both ears of cocci bacteria and yeast found on in-house cytology**. A prescription for **Animax ointment is in the record, for 1" of ointment in both ears BID × 10 days**. This can be dispensed from the hospital.

A **recheck for the ears and booster vaccines** will need to be scheduled **for 4 weeks**.

You need to fill in the template in the electronic medical record before Ms. Kulwicki can be checked out.

Directions: Indicate what bolded information will be entered into the various areas of a POMR medical record. Complete the prescription label for both the Simparica Trio and the Animax ointment.

PROBLEM-ORIENTED MEDICAL RECORD

Defined database

Master problem list

Plan

Progress

    Subjective

    Objective

    Assessment

    Plan

PRESCRIPTION LABEL SIMPARICA

Guthry Animal Hospital
Doctor Guthry

Client name:

Patient name:

Date: 1/1/01

Rx:

Medication name:

Directions:

Amount:

Refills:

Keep out of reach of children. For veterinary use only!

PRESCRIPTION LABEL ANIMAX

Guthry Animal Hospital
Doctor Guthry

Client name:

Patient name:

Date: 1/1/01

Rx:

Medication name:

Directions:

Amount:

Refills:

Keep out of reach of children. For veterinary use only!

3 Medical Terminology

DEFINITIONS

Give the meaning of the following word parts.

1. ex- _____

2. hyper- _____

3. pre- _____

4. dis- _____

5. dys- _____

6. -gram _____

7. cardi- _____

8. peri- _____

9. -ectomy _____

10. tachy- _____

11. -rrhea _____

12. -pathy _____

13. -pexy _____

14. -plasia _____

15. -oma _____

16. -osis _____

17. -itis _____

18. -megaly _____

19. -tome _____

20. poly- _____

MATCHING

Match the meaning with the prefix or suffix.

1. _____ -megaly	A. against
2. _____ hypo-	B. inflammation
3. _____ hydro-	C. hidden
4. _____ glycol-	D. abnormal state or condition
5. _____ -eu	E. enlargement
6. _____ anti-	F. slow
7. _____ -ize	G. normal
8. _____ -itis	H. sweet
9. _____ brady-	I. difficult
10. _____ -osis	J. use, subject to
11. _____ dys-	K. water
12. _____ -crypt	L. insufficient

Give the correct medical term for each.

1. Before birth _____

2. Little urine _____

3. Excessive eating _____

4. Difficult breathing _____

5. Excessively slow heart rate _____

6. Out of place _____

7. Pertaining to throughout the entire animal kingdom _____

8. Not enough red blood cells _____

9. Difficulty swallowing _____

10. New tissue growth _____

11. Examination of a dead animal _____

12. Inability to move one side of the body _____

13. Long headed _____

14. Study of the endocrine system _____

15. Sugar in the urine _____

16. Inducing death painlessly _____

17. To make free from infection _____

18. Excessively fast heart rate _____

19. The plural of phalanx _____

20. Body temperature higher than normal _____

1. The term for toward the midline is:
   a. medial
   b. lateral
   c. proximal
   d. distal

2. The paw is _____ to the shoulder.
   a. cranial
   b. caudal
   c. distal
   d. proximal

3. What is the meaning of the suffix -plasty?
   a. excision
   b. forming an opening
   c. surgical repair
   d. incision

4. Which term describes an incision into the duodenum?
   a. duodenectomy
   b. duodenoscopy
   c. duodenostomy
   d. duodenotomy

5. Which terms pertain to the tongue?
   a. lingual and gingival
   b. lingual and glossal
   c. lingual only
   d. gingival and glossal

6. Cystotomy is:
   a. resection of the urinary bladder
   b. incision into the urinary bladder
   c. inflammation of the urinary bladder
   d. herniation of the urinary bladder

7. Polyuria:
   a. is an abbreviated way of saying renal failure
   b. is the opposite of anuria
   c. means having more than one kidney
   d. means having multiple pouches developing from the urinary bladder

8. Nephromegaly is:
   a. inflammation of the kidney
   b. suturing of the kidney
   c. constriction of the kidney
   d. enlargement of the kidney

9. Which term refers to nasal discharge?
   a. rhinitis
   b. rhinorrhea
   c. rhinorrhagia
   d. epistaxis

10. Which term describes the surgical incision into the chest wall?
    a. thoracentesis
    b. thoracostomy
    c. thoracotomy
    d. thoracectomy

11. Which term describes a benign growth of fat cells?
    a. lipoma
    b. liposarcoma
    c. adipocarcinoma
    d. adiposarcoma

12. Which term describes dead tissue?
    a. necrotic
    b. plantigrade
    c. polled
    d. exfoliative

13. Which term describes the removal of the thyroid gland?
    a. thyroidotomy
    b. thyroidectomy
    c. thyroplasty
    d. thyroplegia

14. Which term describes a disease of the adrenal glands?
    a. adrenal pathogen
    b. adrenopathy
    c. adenopathy
    d. adenosis

15. What is the plural of stimulus?
    a. stimulum
    b. stimulae
    c. stimula
    d. stimuli

16. The term *ectopic* means:
    a. in the usual location
    b. outside the usual place
    c. outside the uterus
    d. outside the reproductive system

17. Which term describes inflammation of the outer ear?
    a. otitis externa
    b. otitis media
    c. otitis interna
    d. panotitis

18. Which prefix means "down, under, lower, against"?
    a. cata-
    b. andro-
    c. ana-
    d. cart-

19. Which of the following suggests "lesser, decreased"?
    a. hyper-
    b. super-
    c. hypo-
    d. ultra-

20. Which of the following terms means an instrument for cutting bone?
    a. osteotomy
    b. osteotome
    c. arthroscopy
    d. arthroscope

21. Which of the following terms means paralysis of one side of the body?
    a. hemodynia
    b. hemiplegia
    c. holomegaly
    d. holorrhexis

22. Which of the following terms means a suture fixating the stomach?
    a. gastroplasty
    b. gastropexy
    c. gastrorrhaphy
    d. cystomegaly

23. The term *nephrotomy* means:
    a. surgical removal of the kidneys
    b. a mouthlike opening into the kidneys
    c. cutting into the kidneys
    d. visual examination of the kidneys

24. *Dysuria* means:
    a. deficient urine production
    b. painful or difficult urination
    c. blood in the urine
    d. pertaining to urination

25. *Polyphagia* means:
    a. decreased hunger
    b. excessive eating
    c. no eating
    d. much drinking

26. Which of the following is most likely to be seen in a cat diagnosed with a bacterial urinary tract infection?
    a. anuria
    b. oliguria
    c. pyuria
    d. nocturia

27. *Osteoarthropathy* means:
    a. disease of the bone and joint
    b. surgical removal of the bone and cartilage
    c. infection of the bone and joint
    d. destruction of the bone and cartilage

28. Which of the following means surgical removal of the gall bladder?
    a. cholecystectomy
    b. cystocentesis
    c. cholecystoplasty
    d. cholecystemia

29. *Cystocentesis* means:
    a. movement of the thorax
    b. sensation of the bladder
    c. abnormal condition of the abdomen
    d. surgical puncture of the bladder

30. Which one of the following terms is in the plural form?
    a. testis
    b. testes
    c. granuloma
    d. appendix

31. What term describes an abnormally rapid respiratory rate?
    a. apnea
    b. bradypnea
    c. dyspnea
    d. tachypnea

32. *Polyuria* means:
    a. decreased urine production
    b. blood in the urine
    c. pain in the urethra
    d. much urine

33. Which term describes the machine that records electrical impulses from the heart?
    a. electrocardiogram
    b. cardiometer
    c. cardioscope
    d. electrocardiograph

34. Which of the following terms means paralysis of the eye?
    a. oculoplegia
    b. ophthalmoparesis
    c. otopexy
    d. blepharoptosis

35. *Peritoneal* means:
    a. pertaining to the peritoneum
    b. a condition of the periosteum
    c. inflammation of the peritoneum
    d. a disease of the periosteum

36. What term describes the procedure in which a laparoscope is used to view the abdominal cavity?
    a. abdominoscopy
    b. abdominometry
    c. laparoscopy
    d. laparotomy

37. Which of the following terms means disease of the hair?
    a. trichopathy
    b. pilosis
    c. tracheoplasty
    d. pilosclerosis

38. *Myositis* means:
    a. inflammation of the muscles
    b. inflammation of the spinal cord
    c. a condition of the muscles
    d. a condition of the spinal cord

39. Pertaining to the cranium or head end of the body
    a. cardio-
    b. cysto-
    c. crani-
    d. costo-

40. Pertains to the undersurface of the rear foot
    a. plantar
    b. palmar
    c. ventro
    d. dorso

41. The chewing or biting surface of teeth
    a. buccal
    b. lingual
    c. contact
    d. occlusal

42. The act of bending, such as a joint
    a. flexion
    b. abduction
    c. adduction
    d. extension

43. Pertaining to the underside of a quadruped
    a. ventral
    b. dorsal
    c. medial
    d. lateral

44. Pertaining to the back or top area of a body
    a. ventral
    b. dorsal
    c. medial
    d. lateral

45. Toward the cheek
    a. mesial
    b. lingual
    c. buccal
    d. occlusal

46. Lying face up
    a. supine
    b. prone
    c. ventral
    d. dorsal

47. Denoting a position farther from the median plane of the body
    a. proximal
    b. distal
    c. abduction
    d. adduction

48. Movement of a limb or part away from the median line
    a. proximal
    b. distal
    c. abduction
    d. adduction

49. The act of straightening
    a. extension
    b. flexion
    c. medial
    d. proximal

50. Pertaining to the tail end of the body
    a. cranial
    b. caudal
    c. mesial
    d. dorsal

17

MATCHING ABBREVIATIONS

1. BAR _____	a) Four times a day
2. bid _____	b) As often as needed
3. dx _____	c) Bright, alert, responsive
4. FLUTD _____	d) Intramuscular
5. rx _____	e) Diagnosis
6. GI _____	f) Feline lower urinary tract disease
7. HBC _____	g) History
8. hx _____	h) Physical examination
9. IM _____	i) Gastrointestinal
10. IV _____	j) Fracture
11. MM _____	k) Hit by car
12. NM _____	l) Treatment
13. PE _____	m) Intravenous
14. PO _____	n) Neutered male
15. PRN _____	o) By mouth
16. PU/PD _____	p) Polyuria/polydipsia
17. qid _____	q) Once a day
18. SF _____	r) Subcutaneous
19. SC _____	s) Temperature, pulse, respiration
20. sid _____	t) Three times a day
21. tid _____	u) Mucous membrane
22. TPR _____	v) Twice a day
23. tx _____	w) Upper respiratory infection
24. URI _____	x) Urinary tract infection
25. UTI _____	y) Spayed female
26. fx _____	z) Prescription

CASE SCENARIO

You have received records for one of your clients seen by the local emergency Clinic for an HBC. These records have a lot of words you are not exactly familiar with.

Referring Clinic: All Creatures Veterinary Hospital, PC

Referring Veterinarian: Dr. C. Palmer

Client: Jeffery, Sophia

Patient: Malcolm

Presenting complaint: 7 yr old **NM**(1) **K9**(2) English Bulldog (**brachycephalic**) (3) reportedly **HBC**(4) while out for a walk with (5)**O** ~30 min ago. Malcolm was grazed by a passing sedan and sustained a (6) **superficial** wound to the (7)**cranial**, (8) **dorsal** aspect of the (9) (10) **thoracocervico** area

(11)**PE**:

    Subjective:
        Body condition score (BCS): 3/5
        Pain score: 4/5
        No (12) **Platelets** (13)**CNS** deficits detected
        (14) **MM** pale with a 3 second capillary refill time

        (15) **Diarrhea** found along caudal rear legs

    Objective:
        T: 103.5 (16) (**hyperthermia**)
        P: 180 (17) **bpm** (**tachycardia**)
        R: 100 (18) **bpm** (**tachypnea**)
        (19) **BW**: 65# (29.5 kg)

(20)**Dx** Tests:
        (21) **CBC**: (22) **PCV** − 25% ((23) **RBC** decreased, showing signs of mild (24) **anemia**). (25) **WBC** within normal limits. (26) Platelets- adequate
        (27) **Glucometer**: 180 mg/dl (28) (**hyperglycemia**)
        Radiographs: (29) **lateral and** (30) **ventral dorsal** (v/d) thorax and abdominal rads.
        Thoracic films: no evidence of (31) **fx** ribs, some (32) **SC** emphysema seen as air pockets under the skin. Swelling and (33) **dermatitis** present from rib spaces #3-#7.
        Abdominal films: The diaphragm appears intact with no signs of organ displacement. Air present in (34) **caudal** stomach, and (35) **cranial** duodenum. The bladder is intact and full.
        (36) **Electrocardiogram** (ECG): Normal sinus rhythm, with significant (37) **tachycardia** present

        (38) **UA**: 10 ml of urine collected by (39) **cystocentesis**. Urinalysis- no significant findings. (40) **SG** 1.035

(41) **Tx**:
        IV catheter: 20 ga (42) **peripheral** catheter placed in the (43) **distal** 1/3rd of the RF leg, (44) **proximal** to the carpus
        Fluid bolus LRS @ 120 ml/hr x 12 hours: 1440 mls (45) **IV**
        Morphine @ 2 mg/kg (46) (47) **IM qid** (10 mg/ml): 59 mg, 5.9 mls IM
        Carprofen @ 4.4 mg/kg (48) (49) **SC bid** (50 mg/ml): 130 mg (129.8 mg), 2.6 mls SC
        Debride wound to the (50) **dorsal** surface of thorax: All injuries are (51) **superficial**. Injured area flushed well with 0.9% saline until all debris was flushed out.
        Non-adherent bandage applied to (52) **cranial thorax**: (2) 3 x 3 pads were used to cover the debrided area. (53) **Cranial thorax** wrapped with 3" vet wrap.
    Follow-up recommendation:
        Recheck with referring DVM within 12 hrs
        (54) **Rx:** Carprofen tablets: 100 mg (55) **po bid** x 5 days
        All wounds to heal by second intention
        Change bandage (56) **sid/ q 24 hr**
        Monitor wound for signs of infection
        Monitor for tissue (57) **necrosis** and remove as needed
        Monitor (58) **anemia**
        (59) **Antibiotics** not dispensed pending signs of infection

Provide a definition for all bolded words in this history.

1. _____
2. _____
3. _____
4. _____
5. _____
6. _____
7. _____
8. _____
9. _____
10. _____
11. _____
12. _____
13. _____

14. _____
15. _____
16. _____
17. _____
18. _____
19. _____
20. _____
21. _____
22. _____
23. _____
24. _____
25. _____
26. _____

27. _____

28. _____

29. _____

30. _____

31. _____

32. _____

33. _____

34. _____

35. _____

36. _____

37. _____

38. _____

39. _____

40. _____

41. _____

42. _____

43. _____

44. _____

45. _____

46. _____

47. _____

48. _____

49. _____

50. _____

51. _____

52. _____

53. _____

54. _____

55. _____

56. _____

57. _____

58. _____

59. _____

4 Animal Behavior and Restraint

LEARNING OBJECTIVES

After reviewing this chapter, the reader will be able to:

- Describe the processes by which behaviors develop.
- Differentiate between positive and negative reinforcement and punishment.
- List and describe types of aggressive behavior that may be seen in dogs and cats.
- Describe the role of veterinary professionals in preventing behavior problems.
- List the steps in house-training a puppy.
- Describe proper litter box care.
- List the different options cats look for in scratching posts.
- Describe the role of veterinary professionals in managing behavior problems.
- List and give examples of various behavior modification techniques.
- Describe the procedure for referring clients to professionals for resolution of behavior problems.
- Describe the psychological principles underlying physical restraint techniques.
- Explain and implement the safety precautions taken before and during physical restraint.
- Restrain dogs and cats for routine procedures such as physical examinations, nursing care, and sample collection.
- Give examples of behavior responses of animals to physical restraint.
- Correctly identify and use restraint equipment.

FILL IN THE BLANK

1. For any behavior to occur, there must be a _____.

2. Some problem behaviors are caused by _____ or _____ amounts of neurotransmitters.

3. The study of animal behavior is _____.

4. _____ conditioning refers to the association of stimuli that occur at approximately the same time or in roughly the same area.

5. _____ conditioning refers to the association of a particular activity with a punishment or reward.

6. The most important time period for behavior development in dogs and cats is _____ _____ to _____ weeks of age.

7. Genetics can play a role in behavior problems, but _____ can also cause inappropriate behavior.

8. _____ reinforcement refers to any pleasant occurrence that immediately follows a behavior.

9. _____ and _____ are examples of positive punishment.

10. _____ is any stimulus that decreases the likelihood of a behavior being repeated.

11. Positive punishment involves adding an _____ occurrence to decrease a behavior.

12. _____ punishment involves removing a desirable occurrence to decrease a behavior.

13. A delay of longer than _____ seconds between the behavior and the subsequent reinforcement significantly decreases the effectiveness of the reinforcement.

14. _____ refers to the attribution of human characteristics and emotions to animals.

15. Full house training should not be expected before _____ to _____ months of age.

16. One of the most important motivations for cats that scratch objects with their front claws is _____ marking.

17. The most common complaint from dog owners is aggression toward _____, whereas the most common complaint from cat owners is aggression toward other _____.

18. The sensitive socialization period in cats is _____ to _____ weeks.

19. In assessing a case of behavior problems, medical conditions that may account for the behavioral signs should first be evaluated; this is especially important with _____ and _____.

20. Behavior modification is needed to accompany _____ to increase the chances of a successful resolution of the problem.

Match the breed name with the correct image.

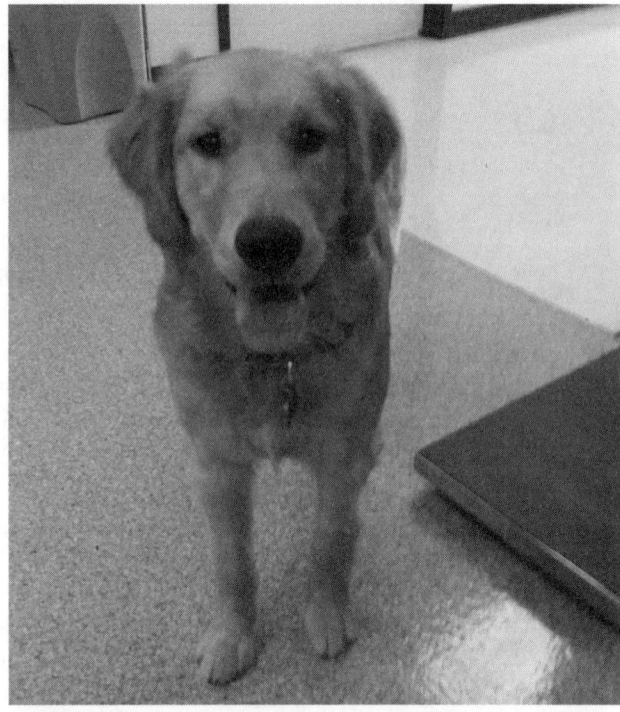

a. Papillon

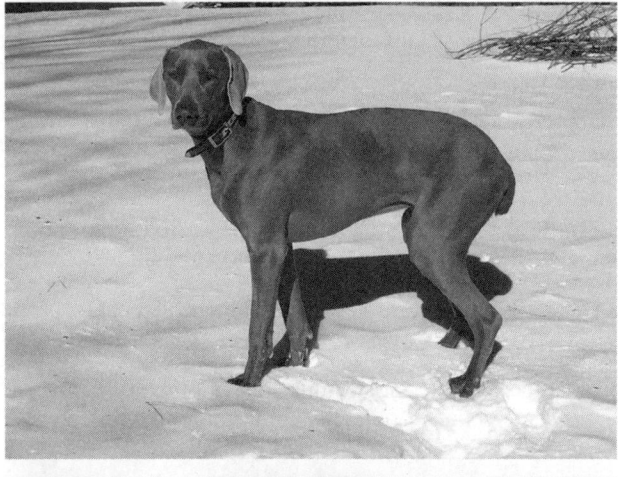

b. Beagle

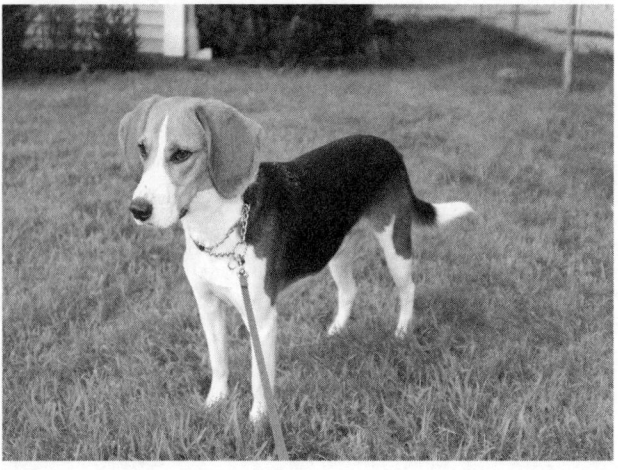

c. French Bulldog

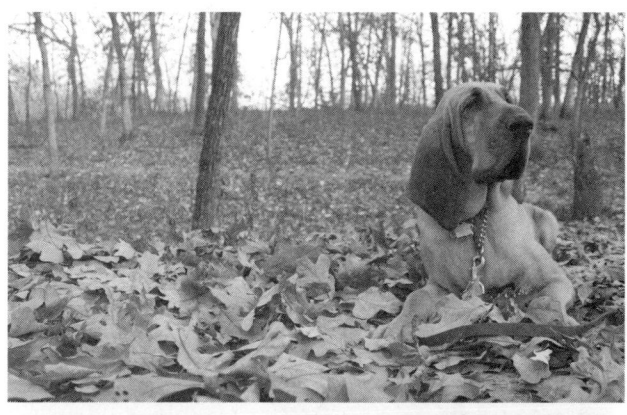

d. Australian Shepherd

e. Bloodhound

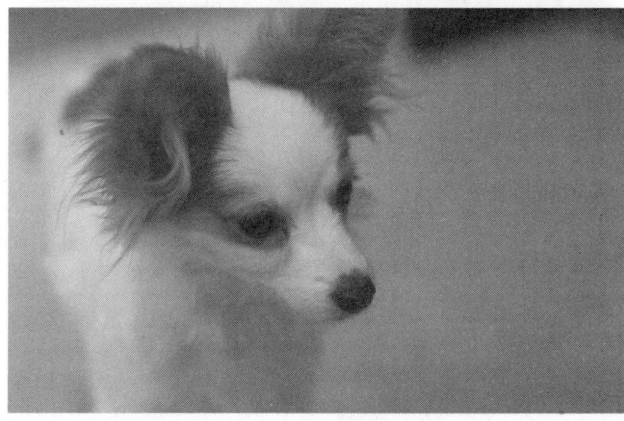

f. Weimaraner

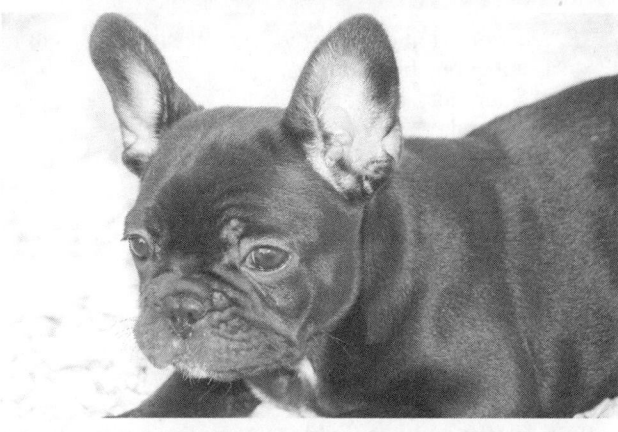

g. Shetland Sheepdog

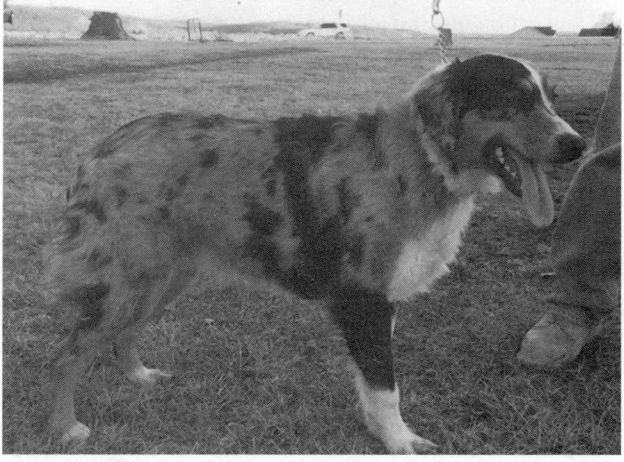

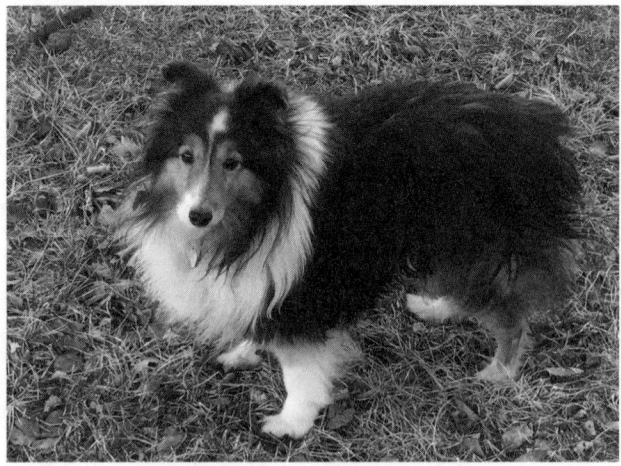

h. Golden Retriever

MULTIPLE CHOICE

1. What are veterinarians who meet the established criteria set by the American College of Veterinary Behavior called?
   a. Board certified
   b. Licensed
   c. Registered
   d. Technicians

2. Through which process was the developement of different breeds of animals done?
   a. Socialization
   b. Selective breeding
   c. Entrapment
   d. Imprinting

3. Which organization maintains a database of dog breeds?
   a. AAFP
   b. ACVB
   c. USDA
   d. AKC

4. What piece of equipment can be used to prevent a fearful dog from biting?
   a. Restrain pole
   b. Slip leash
   c. Muzzle
   d. Gauntlets

5. What body position can be used to perform a routine physical examination on a cat?
   a. Sternal
   b. Dorsal
   c. Palmar
   d. Plantar

6. When restraining a cat, how is it determined how much restraint is required?
   a. Always approach every cat with the maximum force you are capable of
   b. Scruffing will control all cats, every time
   c. All cats need to be placed inside a restraint bag
   d. Use the minimal amount of restraint needed to get the job done

7. What position is preferred when positioning a cat for a saphenous blood draw?
   a. Standing
   b. Lateral
   c. Dorsal
   d. Sternal

8. When holding a dog for a standing restraint, where do they need to be positioned?
   a. Within arm's reach
   b. Far away from your body
   c. Close to the doctor
   d. Close to you

9. Sometimes it is possible to complete a procedure on a cat by puffing air in the animal's face. What kind of technique is this?
   a. Muzzling
   b. Distraction
   c. Dominance
   d. Passive

10. What type of aggression is most commonly seen at the hospital?
    a. Territorial
    b. Maternal
    c. Dominance
    d. Fearful

11. What type of aggression do owners report most at home with cats?
    a. Toward children
    b. Between cats
    c. Territorial
    d. Maternal

12. Which organization maintains a database of cat breeds?
    a. AKC
    b. ICA
    c. DEA
    d. AVBP

13. When is the primary socialization period for puppies?
    a. Birth–4 weeks
    b. 2–7 weeks
    c. 3–12 weeks
    d. 16–24 weeks

14. Fear-free practices look at decreasingwhat kind of response?
    a. FAS
    b. Socialization
    c. Negative conditioning
    d. Innate

15. What type of conditioning can reinforce good behavior?
    a. Imprinting
    b. Pecking order
    c. Operant
    d. Classical

16. Which conditioning is an example of withholding attention from a jumping dog?
    a. Negative punishment
    b. Classical
    c. Positive reinforcement
    d. Aversives

17. What type of aggression is directed toward humans who are not members of the family?
    a. Pain induced
    b. Maternal
    c. Predatory
    d. Territorial

18. What is the leading cause for dogs and cats being surrendered or euthanized?
    a. Poor training retention
    b. Behavioral problems
    c. Not being able to afford expensive surgeries
    d. They do not match the new flooring

19. Anthropomorphism refers to what kind of behavior?
    a. Aggression between unneutered males
    b. Eating their food too fast causing vomiting
    c. The attribution of human characteristics and emotions to animals
    d. Attachment of very young animals to humans

20. What physical changes must occur before puppies can become house trained?
    a. Core strength
    b. 50% of anticipated adult size
    c. Sexual maturity
    d. Social maturity

21. Under what conditions do most "accidents" with puppies occur?
    a. They are being spiteful
    b. They are unsupervised
    c. After neutering
    d. It is cold outside

22. Crate training a puppy can help with what types of behaviors?
    a. Innate
    b. Play
    c. Territorial
    d. Destructive

23. What type of reinforcement can be helpful when house-training a puppy?
    a. Clicker
    b. Spanking
    c. Isolation
    d. Pointing out the accident and rubbing their noses in it

24. Use of a litter box with cats is what type of behavior?
    a. Learned from the Queen
    b. Taught by the owners
    c. Environmentally reinforced
    d. Instinctual

25. The preferred substrate in litter boxes for cats is what material?
    a. Cats have no preference and will use whatever material is given to them
    b. Litters with floral scents
    c. Fine-grained clumping litter
    d. Organic, easily compostable litter

26. In a household with two cats, it is recommended that there be how many litter boxes?
    a. 1
    b. 2
    c. 3
    d. 4

27. What is one of the most important motivators for cats scratching objects with their front feet?
    a. Territorial marking
    b. Wanton destruction
    c. Stimulating their appetites
    d. Burning calories

28. What is one of the most overlooked features when selecting a scratching post?
    a. Cost
    b. Construction materials
    c. Height
    d. Weight

29. When should a well-worn, torn-up scratching post be replaced?
    a. Yearly
    b. When they become unsightly
    c. At the first sign of damage
    d. When they are dangerous to the cat

30. What should the owner do if a dog is caught chewing an unacceptable item?
    a. Spank the dog firmly
    b. Take it away and replace it with an acceptable toy
    c. Yell in a firm voice
    d. Take away all of the toys

31. What type of behavior is seen in situations involving social conflict?
    a. Agnostic
    b. Atheists
    c. Innate
    d. Destructive

32. When dealing with a fearful or aggressive dog, what changes in your body posture should you do?
    a. Approach them head-on, looking directly at them
    b. Never approach and use a restraint pole
    c. Avoid looking directly at them and turn your body sideways
    d. Sit on the floor so you are at their eye level and lower your head

33. What is the easiest and safest way to remove a small, friendly dog from a cage?
    a. Grasp gently around the chest and lift out
    b. Throw a slip leash over their head and use this to lower them to the floor
    c. Open the door and let them jump out
    d. Slip a muzzle over their noses and cover them with a large towel

34. When selecting an Elizabethan collar to use on a dog, what would be the correct length?
    a. It comes within an inch of the end of the dog's muzzle
    b. It is the same length as the dog's muzzle
    c. It extends past the end of the nose
    d. As long as it fits around the neck, the length is not important

35. When restraining a pregnant bitch, what do you need to be aware of?
    a. To hold the dog as close to you as possible
    b. To not apply too much pressure around her abdomen
    c. To control all four legs
    d. A firm scruff works very well during pregnancy

36. What information is used to determine an animal's FAS level?
    a. Body posture and vocalization
    b. Appetite and hydration
    c. Heart rate and pulse rates
    d. Vaccine status and type of heartworm prevention used

37. For an animal who is actively lunging at you, what restraint options are available to minimize your chances of being bitten?
    a. A gauze muzzle followed by a nylon muzzle
    b. A big fluffy towel and gauntlets
    c. An Elizabethan collar
    d. A restraint pole

38. A dog whose tail is up and wagging, actively seeking attention, while accepting treats from you would have what level of FAS?
    a. 0
    b. 1
    c. 2
    d. 3

39. When approaching a newborn litter of puppies with their mom, what type of behavior would be expected?
    a. Agnostic
    b. Territorial
    c. Aggressive
    d. Maternal

40. What would be an appropriate restraint device for a dog with an FAS of 3 with the potential to bite?
    a. Slip leash
    b. Close body hug
    c. Gauntlets
    d. Muzzle

41. An animal who is lying on their belly, with their chest in full contact with the floor/table, is in what position?
    a. Sternal
    b. Dorsal
    c. Lateral
    d. Standing

42. A technique that uses food or other treats to direct the animal away from a procedure that is being done.
    a. Aversion
    b. Pain
    c. Distraction
    d. Sedation

43. What is the state called when an animal is being physically constrained?
    a. Sedation
    b. Aversion
    c. Restraint
    d. Distraction

44. Which term describes a dog's expression, exhibited by having ears drawn down and back, showing white around the pupils of the eyes, not making any eye contact, and cowering?
    a. Relaxed
    b. Fearful
    c. Distracted
    d. Aggressive

45. To encourage a cat to play with or use an object, it can be sprayed or rubbed with catnip or a what type of commercial scent?
    a. Disinfectant
    b. Pheromone
    c. Essential oils
    d. Odor blocking

46. What is the most common behavioral problem with pet birds?
    a. Biting
    b. Throwing their food around
    c. Destroying their perches
    d. Flying into ceiling fans

47. A stimulus is defined as what type of response?
    a. Any action performed by an animal
    b. An internal or external change that exceeds a threshold, causing stimulation of the nervous or endocrine system
    c. The study of animal behavior, excluding humans
    d. The association of a particular activity with a punishment or reward

48. What is a rapid learning process that enables a newborn animal to recognize and bond with its caretaker?
    a. Imprinting
    b. Operant conditioning
    c. Positive reinforcement
    d. Ethology

49. The study of animal behavior
    a. Biology
    b. Ethology
    c. Behaviorology
    d. Technology

50. Exposure of a young animal to new experiences, people, other animals, and places with the goal of preventing fearful or anxious behavior as adults.
    a. Neutering
    b. Situational
    c. Socialization
    d. Scent marking

CASE SCENARIO

Because of your interest in behavior, Dr. Kennedy has asked you to update the new puppy and kitten handout that the clinic gives to new clients.

She wants you to include information on house training/litter box use, early socialization, and helpful tips and tricks.

Fill in the forms below to give to Dr. Kennedy.

New Puppy Information

Age	Behavior	Reinforcers
2 months- _____ months	House training	1. _____ 2. _____ 3. _____ 4. _____ 5. _____
3 weeks- the life of the animal	Early socialization	1. _____ 2. _____ 3. _____ 4. _____ 5. _____ 6. _____

Age	Behavior	Reinforcers
	Helpful tips	1. _____
		2. _____
		3. _____
		4. _____
		5. _____
		6. _____
		7. _____

New Kitten Information

Age	Behavior	Reinforcers
Kittens- adults	Litterbox training	1. _____
		2. _____
		3. _____
		4. _____
		5. _____
		6. _____
3 weeks- the life of the animal	Early socialization	1. _____
		2. _____
		3. _____
		4. _____
		5. _____
	Cat-trees and Scratching posts	1. _____
		2. _____
		3. _____
	Helpful tips	1. _____
		2. _____
		3. _____
		4. _____
		5. _____
		6. _____
		7. _____

5 Animal Husbandry and Nutrition

LEARNING OBJECTIVES

After reviewing this chapter, the reader will be able to:

- Discuss features of appropriate housing and nutrition for animals.
- Discuss general housekeeping concerns in the veterinary practice.
- Explain the principles of sanitation that relate to disease prevention.
- List basic energy-producing and non–energy-producing nutrients.
- Describe considerations for feeding young and adult dogs.
- Describe considerations for feeding young and adult cats.
- Discuss the fundamentals of exotic pet diet considerations.
- List and describe common diseases and ways in which they can affect people.
- Discuss methods used to control the spread of zoonotic diseases.
- Explain the general principles underlying disease prevention.
- List and discuss types of vaccinations and schedules of vaccinations for domestic animal species.
- Describe factors that predispose to disease.

FILL IN THE BLANK

1. An agent that causes an abnormal increase in body temperature is a _____.

2. Water balance in the system affects the ability to excrete _____.

3. After an anorexic patient has had a feeding tube placed, food is initially started at _____% DER.

4. Allowing pets free access to food at any time increases _____, which leads to obesity.

5. Which association developed nutritional standards for pet food production? _____.

6. Sick or injured pets need good nutritional support to counteract the immunosuppressive effects of _____, _____, _____, _____, and _____.

7. All enteral feeding tube diets should be administered at _____ to _____.

8. Evaluating tissues with a microscope is called _____.

9. Water-soluble vitamins are passively absorbed from the _____.

10. Cats require _____ fatty acids in their diet.

11. Husbandry involves _____, _____, and _____ of animals.

12. The ambient room temperature in the veterinary environment should be kept at _____ to _____.

13. The general rule for a holding enclosure is a minimum of _____ times the body size of the animal.

14. _____ is the destruction of microorganisms or their toxins.

15. A ventilation system should be capable of exhausting all air within a building in _____ to _____ minutes to facilitate odor control.

16. A _____ is any constituent of food that is ingested to support life.

17. Two means of controlling the intake of a pet's food are _____ and _____ control.

18. The most common form of malnutrition in pets is _____.

19. The end result of tissue repair is usually _____ or _____.

20. Highly vascularized connective tissue produced after extensive tissue damage is called _____ tissue.

21. Organisms that can cause disease in a host are _____.

22. Bacteria are classified either as _____ or _____.

23. Diseases transmitted between animals and people are _____ diseases.

24. The infective agent in 50% of dog bites and 90% of cat bites is _____.

25. Cat bites are _____ more times likely to become infected than dog bites.

26. A sign of anal sacculitis is _____ _____.

27. Inappropriate urination is one symptom of _____.

28. Swelling and a rapidly growing firm mass at the site of a recent vaccination in a cat are common signs of _____.

29. Chronic infections of the oral cavity, skin, and respiratory tract; chronic fever; and cachexia in a cat are common signs of _____.

30. One sign of infectious canine tracheobronchitis (kennel cough) is _____.

MATCHING

Match the following items with the descriptions.

1. _____ Body-conditioning score	A. Amino acid that is synthesized in the body
2. _____ Forage	B. Meat eater
3. _____ Fat-soluble vitamins	C. Vitamins absorbed from the small intestines—excess amount excreted in urine
4. _____ Herbivore	D. Vitamins metabolized and stored in the liver
5. _____ Obesity	E. Plant eater
6. _____ Portion-control feeding	F. Method of subjectively qualifying body fat reserves
7. _____ Free-choice feeding	G. Portion fed with access for only 10–15 minutes
8. _____ Time-control feeding	H. Daily portion offered either in a single feeding or divided into several portions
9. _____ Water	I. Foundation for metabolism of all nutrients in the body
10. _____ Essential amino acids	J. Most common nutritional disorder of pets
11. _____ Nonessential amino acids	K. Feeds made up of most or all plant
12. _____ Nutrient	L. Access to food 24 hours a day
13. _____ Carnivore	M. Amino acid that cannot be synthesized in the body
14. _____ Water-soluble vitamins	N. Any constituent of food that can be ingested to support life

LISTS EXPLANATIONS

1. List the six basic nutrients:
   1. _____
   2. _____
   3. _____
   4. _____
   5. _____
   6. _____

2. Name five dietary minerals named in this chapter:
   1. _____
   2. _____
   3. _____
   4. _____
   5. _____

3. List the fat-soluble vitamins:
   1. _____
   2. _____
   3. _____
   4. _____

4. Obesity may predispose pets to what three things?
   1. _____
   2. _____
   3. _____

5. Describe techniques used to enhance the aroma and taste of food for cats:
   1. _____
   2. _____
   3. _____
   4. _____

6. Name three reasons that homemade diets are not always the best for a pet:
   1. _____
   2. _____
   3. _____

7. What does the acronym AAFCO stand for?
   _____

8. List the water-soluble vitamins:
   1. _____
   2. _____
   3. _____
   4. _____

9. A hospitalized patient is a candidate for nutritional support if the following occurs:
   1. _____
   2. _____
   3. _____

10. List the classifications of carbohydrates:
   1. _____
   2. _____
   3. _____

MULTIPLE CHOICE

1. Which of the following is not an essential fatty acid in cats?
   a. linoleic
   b. linolenic
   c. taurine
   d. arachidonic

2. What is energy used for?
   a. metabolism
   b. fighting disease
   c. skin turgor
   d. clotting

3. What is dietary protein used for?
   a. digestion
   b. metabolism
   c. building body tissue
   d. cell repair

4. In regard to cow's milk which nutrients are found in inappropriate levels for neonatal puppies?
   a. glucose and phosphorus
   b. protein and lactose
   c. potassium and sodium
   d. iron and selenium

5. What components are needed in enhanced levels in diets for active dogs?
   a. magnesium
   b. selenium
   c. fat
   d. phosphorus

6. Under which condition(s) would a patient be a candidate for nutritional support?
   a. lost more than 10% of body weight
   b. diarrhea with body-conditioning loss
   c. organ dysfunction
   d. all of the above

7. Which route is used for enteral nutritional support?
   a. oral
   b. parenteral
   c. intravenous
   d. subcutaneous

8. What is responsible for the digestion of cellulose fiber in herbivores?
   a. Lactase and amylase
   b. Bacteria found in the stomach or hindgut
   c. Protozoa and fungi
   d. Genetic modifications to the intestinal villi

9. Which organic compound is made of chains of amino acids?
   a. fatty acids
   b. complex carbohydrates
   c. nondigestible fibers
   d. proteins

10. Which nutrient contains more energy per unit of weight than any other?
   a. water
   b. carbohydrates
   c. fats
   d. proteins

11. Which nutrients are essential for life but provide no calories?
   a. vitamins and minerals
   b. amino acids and proteins
   c. fats and lipids
   d. water and fiber

12. Which of these is *not* an essential mineral?
   a. sodium
   b. chloride
   c. lithium
   d. iron

13. Which of these nutrients is used for energy production?
    a. B-complex vitamins
    b. vitamins A, D, and K
    c. proteins
    d. water

14. Where are fat-soluble vitamins stored after digestion?
    a. liver
    b. kidneys
    c. spleen
    d. bone marrow

15. Nutrition that is provided through a central intravenous catheter is called what?
    a. essential
    b. parenteral
    c. enteral
    d. incomplete

16. A food with a higher biological value has higher levels of what nutrient?
    a. fatty acids
    b. water
    c. amino acids
    d. fiber

17. Which disease in cats is characterized by an excessive accumulation of triglycerides in the liver?
    a. Hepatic lipidosis
    b. Diabetes
    c. Stage 4 CRF
    d. Dilated cardiomyopathy

18. Which mineral is typically limited in diets formulated for use in animals with renal failure?
    a. copper
    b. iron
    c. calcium
    d. phosphorus

19. What nutrient is required for the absorption of the B-complex vitamins?
    a. protein
    b. water
    c. fats
    d. complex carbohydrates

20. Which nutrient can cause toxicities if consumed in excessive amounts?
    a. carbohydrates
    b. water
    c. fat-soluble vitamins
    d. macrominerals

21. What type of amino acids cannot be synthesized in the body and must be supplied by the diet?
    a. conditional
    b. water-soluble
    c. fat-soluble
    d. essential

22. First-intention healing is seen under what circumstances?
    a. surgical wound closure
    b. granulation tissue is present
    c. a dirty wound
    d. infection

23. What is the name for small stones that obstruct the urethra?
    a. choleoliths
    b. trichobezoar
    c. uroliths
    d. renal calculi

24. What term is used to describe diseases transmitted between animals and people?
    a. zoonoses
    b. venereal
    c. direct pathogenesis
    d. antiviral

25. When would a necropsy be performed?
    a. during a spay
    b. after an animal has died
    c. after recovering from anesthesia
    d. before their first set of vaccinations

26. What term is used to describe an organism that can cause disease in a host?
    a. zoonoses
    b. venereal
    c. first-intention
    d. pathogen

27. The type of feeding method in which food is offered at all times so the animal can eat at its leisure.
    a. free-choice
    b. portion-control
    c. timed
    d. measured

28. What type of injury can cause damage with no break in the surface of the tissue?
    a. concussion
    b. bruise
    c. laceration
    d. abrasion

29. What term is used to describe a violent shock or jarring of the tissue?
    a. concussion
    b. bruise
    c. laceration
    d. abrasion

30. What is the destruction of microorganisms and their toxins called?
    a. sanitization
    b. sterilizers
    c. antimicrobial
    d. disinfection

31. What is not a way in which nutrients with hydrocarbon structures can produce energy?
    a. digestion
    b. metabolism
    c. homeostasis
    d. transformation

32. What agent is used to reduce the number of organisms to a safe level?
    a. sanitizer
    b. disinfectant
    c. sterilizer
    d. vaccine

33. What is the most common form of malnutrition seen in pets?
    a. vitamin C deficiency
    b. calcium-phosphorus imbalance
    c. arthritis
    d. obesity

34. What is the protein coat surrounding the genetic material of a virus called?
    a. pathogen
    b. RNA
    c. capsid
    d. toxin

35. What term is used to describe an extremely small, nonliving infectious agent that can cause disease in a wide variety of animals?
    a. bacteria
    b. protozoan
    c. toxin
    d. virus

36. What term describes the study of the cause of disease?
    a. ethology
    b. biology
    c. etiology
    d. pathology

37. Prognosis refers to what part of the disease process?
    a. the immunology
    b. the initial infection
    c. the humoral response
    d. the expected outcome

38. What is the end result of tissue repair?
    a. scarring
    b. full range of motion
    c. fur regrowth
    d. osteoporosis

39. If excessive water-soluble vitamins are consumed, how are they removed from the body?
    a. fat metabolism
    b. they are not absorbed from the intestines until needed
    c. excreted in the urine
    d. bound to bile in the upper gastrointestinal tract

40. What is the most reliable method of animal identification?
    a. collar
    b. tags
    c. air tags
    d. microchip

41. What term describes an infection that is acquired in the hospital?
    a. zoonotic
    b. nosocomial
    c. iatrogenic
    d. commensal

42. Weaning of large-breed dogs is usually complete by what age?
    a. 3–4 weeks
    b. 5–7 weeks
    c. 8–10 weeks
    d. 10–12 weeks

43. What term describes a complex disease characterized by bouts of painful urination with possible urethral obstruction?
    a. Uroliths
    b. Failure to thrive
    c. FLUTD
    d. Obesity

44. Why should chemical floor cleaners not be mixed?
    a. caustic vapors can be produced
    b. they can strip the flooring
    c. they are too effective
    d. resistant bacteria can be formed

45. What changes can be attributed to aging?
    a. Increasing calcium requirements
    b. Diminished sense of taste and smell
    c. Decreased touch sensitivity
    d. Increased protein requirements

46. After what age is the average small to medium-sized dog considered geriatric?
    a. 7 years
    b. 10 years
    c. 12 years
    d. 15 years

47. What is a feeding tube that is placed through the nose and ends in the stomach called?
    a. nasoesophageal
    b. nasogastric
    c. esophageal
    d. PEG

48. What type of immunity occurs when an animal develops antibodies on its own?
    a. active
    b. passive
    c. vaccination
    d. permanent

49. What type of feeding tubes can be used by owners at home?
    a. nasoesophageal
    b. nasogastric
    c. esophagostomy
    d. jejunal

CASE SCENARIO

You are preparing surgical discharge instructions for Casey Jones, a M/N 2-year-old Labrador who came in for an intestinal foreign body, with an intestinal perforation that has caused mild peritonitis. The surgery was performed by Dr. Katherine Janeway.

You are using the hospital's standard template. Fill in the areas that are gray.

Date:	1/1/01		
Veterinarians name:			
Client's name:			
Patient's name:			
Gender:			
Surgical procedure:	Intestinal foreign body removal with anastomosis. Mild peritonitis was found secondary to an intestinal perforation	A culture and sensitivity are done to identify the bacteria. In-house cytology identified gram-positive cocci bacteria	What color and shape are the bacteria that were found?
Feeding instructions:	The patient can be fed ¼ of his regular diet at 6 pm, and again at 9 pm:	If Casey eats 2 cups of food/day, how much can he be offered at each feeding?	_____cups
Activity:	Restrict activity until the sutures are removed in 10-14 days.	Provide 3 suggestions on how to restrict Casey's activity	
Medication:	Cephalexin 500 mg 1 cap po BIDEnrofloxacin 68 mg 1.5-tab po SIDStart both medications tonight with his food.	If both medications are given for 10 days, how many tablets will need to be dispensed?	
Sutures and surgical incision:	Monitor the surgical site for any signs of inflammation or irritation.	What 3 signs that Casey's owners need to look for?	
For a surgical incision, what type of healing is seen?			
Culture and sensitivity results:	Fluid was collected from Casey's abdomen and sent out to determine the bacteria that are causing the peritonitis.	We do not anticipate any problems, as this is not a zoonotic infection.	What does zoonosis mean?

A recheck exam needs to be scheduled for 14 days to remove his suture and check his incision site.	What are signs of adequate healing of an incision site?		
Casey is due for his yearly vaccines; these can be given at the time of his recheck.	What are the core vaccines for a 2-year-old dog?		
Casey is routinely exposed to fleas and ticks while out walking with his owner.	What vaccine can be given to help prevent Lyme disease? How often does this need to be repeated?		

6 Animal Care and Nursing

SHORT ANSWER/FILL IN THE BLANK

1. What are the foundations on which sound medical and nursing interventions are based?
   _____
   _____
   _____

2. What is the key to successful history-taking?
   _____
   _____
   _____

3. Which four methods are used to evaluate patients?
   _____
   _____
   _____

4. What parameters are included in the vital signs?
   _____
   _____
   _____

5. Shock, severe sepsis, severe cardiac insufficiency, multiple organ failure, and poor perfusion secondary to anesthesia or surgery or with low environmental temperatures can result in _____
   _____.

6. List five terms used to describe pulse strength or character.
   _____
   _____
   _____.

7. The patient should be in _____ recumbency and allowed to inhale oxygen during the examination if stressed, to facilitate lung expansion and accurate auscultation.

8. Dyspnea may be manifested by _____ a refusal to lie down _____
   _____.

9. Normal urine output in dogs and cats is _____
   _____
   _____.

10. The anal sacs are emptied with the dog restrained in the _____ position.

11. Signs of ear disease include:
    _____
    _____
    _____

12. An enema introduces fluids into the rectum and also stimulates _____.

13. What types of enemas are contraindicated in cats and small dogs?
    _____
    _____
    _____

14. Subcutaneous (SQ) injections are used for:
    _____
    _____
    _____

15. When is the use of winged infusion (butterfly) catheters most appropriate?
    _____
    _____
    _____

16. Securing the intravenous catheter reduces movement of the catheter in the vessel and can decrease the likelihood of:
    _____
    _____
    _____

17. Nasogastric tubes are inserted through the nares and through the _____ to the _____.

18. _____ _____ is one of the most commonly used supportive measures in veterinary medicine and is an important aspect of virtually every critical care case.

19. _____ wounds contain necrotic tissue and foreign material.

20. Inspiratory stridor can be seen with _____ _____ _____

MULTIPLE CHOICE

1. What condition is described by a disruption of cellular and anatomic functional continuity?
   a. Obesity
   b. Wounds
   c. Disinfection
   d. Surgery

2. Tenesmus is straining to perform what activity?
   a. Eat
   b. Urinate
   c. Defecate
   d. Move

3. What term describes a slower-than-normal heart rate?
   a. Bradycardia
   b. Tachycardia
   c. Bradyarrhythmia
   d. Tachypnea

4. Dehiscence describes what type of surgical wound?
   a. A normal closure
   b. Second-intention closure
   c. Premature opening
   d. Contaminated

5. What tool is used to ensure the nail bed is trimmed down without causing trauma or bleeding?
   a. Kelly hemostat
   b. Rotary grinding tool
   c. Resco trimmer
   d. Styptic powder

6. During euthanasia performed using an injectable barbiturate, death is caused by stopping what process?
   a. Vital life functions
   b. Voluntary muscle activity
   c. Eating
   d. Urination

7. What process is used to clean a contaminated wound?
   a. Percussion
   b. Auscultation
   c. Disinfection
   d. Lavage

8. What type of skin changes can be seen in recumbent patients?
   a. Dehiscence
   b. Decubital ulcers
   c. Degloving wounds
   d. Hemorrhoids

9. Cyanotic mucous membranes can present as what color?
   a. Yellow
   b. Pale pink
   c. Bright red
   d. Blue

10. Which type of topical antibacterial products can impede wound healing the most?
    a. Ointments
    b. Cremes
    c. Water-soluble
    d. Fat-soluble

11. What term describes an abnormally high body temperature?
    a. Hyperthermia
    b. Hypothermia
    c. Hyperfebrile
    d. Hyporexia

12. Which respiratory noise is defined as a low-pitched, snoring noise?
    a. Expiratory dyspnea
    b. Orthopnea
    c. Stridor
    d. Stertor

13. What other route can be used for injectable medications in pediatric patients when an IV catheter is not available?
    a. SQ
    b. IM
    c. ID
    d. IO

14. Which term is used to describe a faster-than-normal respiratory rate?
    a. Tachypnea
    b. Orthopnea
    c. Bradypnea
    d. Dyspnea

15. When rewarming a hypothermic patient, at what time do you stop warming efforts?
    a. 97°F/36°C
    b. 99°F/37°C
    c. 101°F/38°C
    d. 103°F/40°C

16. An animal who is dyspneic if having difficulty doing what?
    a. Urinating
    b. Eating
    c. Defecating
    d. Breathing

17. Which term is used to describe a high-pitched, harsh, wheezy noise?
    a. Stridor
    b. Stertor
    c. Dyspnea
    d. Orthopnea

18. Under what conditions can local anesthetics be used for wound management?
    a. A general anesthetic is unavailable
    b. It is superficial
    c. Surgical debridement
    d. A dirty wound

19. What equipment is preferred when trimming a cat's toenails?
    a. A rotary grinder
    b. White's bypass trimmers
    c. Human toenail trimmers
    d. Resco guillotine trimmers

20. What term describes respiratory distress exacerbated by recumbency?
    a. Orthopnea
    b. Dyspnea
    c. Tachypnea
    d. Stridor

21. This term describes excising dead and dying tissues from around a wound.
    a. Lavage
    b. Auscultation
    c. Debridement
    d. Degloving

22. Auscultation involves using what instrument to listen to sounds produced by the body?
    a. Thermometer
    b. Otoscope
    c. Ophthalmoscope
    d. Stethoscope

23. Peripheral vasoconstriction can cause what change in color to the mucous membranes?
    a. Pale
    b. Brick red
    c. Blue
    d. Yellow

24. What term is used to describe an irregular heartbeat?
    a. Sinus rhythm
    b. Tachycardia
    c. Arrhythmia
    d. Bradycardia

25. What is a normal CRT?
    a. 2 seconds
    b. 102.5°F/39°C
    c. 120 bpm
    d. 15 mL/kg/h

26. Signs of phlebitis include what changes?
    a. Profuse diarrhea and tenesmus
    b. Difficulty urinating, small, frequent urinations
    c. Redness and pain
    d. Profound weight loss, anorexia

27. Which of these is an example of a subnormal body temperature in a cat or dog?
    a. 97°F/36°C
    b. 101°F/38°C
    c. 103°F/40°C
    d. 105°F/41°C

28. What term is used to describe the primary medical problem?
    a. Past medical history
    b. Vaccination status
    c. Presenting complaint
    d. Treatment plan

29. Why is necrotic tissue removed from a wound?
    a. To allow a cosmetic closure
    b. It can act as a growth media for bacteria
    c. It makes bandage application challenging
    d. It continues to drain energy from the animal

30. What is usually the first step in wound management?
    a. Control of bleeding
    b. Lavage
    c. Debridement
    d. Closure

31. Which technique is used to manage hyperthermia?
    a. Ice packs along the belly
    b. Warm water baths
    c. Vasoconstrictive medications
    d. Convective cooling

32. In which age group is ingestion of foreign bodies seen most commonly?
    a. Neonates
    b. Young
    c. Seniors
    d. Neutered

33. What treatment is designed to gently cleanse a wound?
    a. Hemostasis
    b. Lavage
    c. Percussion
    d. Decubital

34. Which description describes regurgitation?
    a. It is passive
    b. It involves straining
    c. Digested food and bile are produced
    d. Aspiration is uncommon

35. Which route of medication administration has the quickest absorption?
    a. Topical
    b. Oral
    c. Subcutaneous
    d. Intravenous

36. Silver nitrate is used for what purpose?
    a. Cauterize quicked nails
    b. Debride wounds
    c. Stimulate respiration
    d. Lower elevated body temperature

37. What is the normal heart rate for cats?
    a. 70–160
    b. 130–325
    c. 150–210
    d. 230–280

38. What type of arrhythmia is normal and affected by breathing?
    a. Respiratory sinus
    b. Acidotic expiration
    c. Bradyarrhythmia
    d. Pulse deficit

39. Over what arteries is pulse quality assessed?
    a. Cephalic
    b. Dorsal pedal
    c. Jugular
    d. Ventral carotid

40. What type of murmurs are often transient and disappear by 3–4 months of age?
    a. Congenital
    b. Physiologic
    c. Anemic
    d. Innocent

41. The normal respiratory rate in dogs is approximately how many beats per minute?
    a. 8–20
    b. 35–60
    c. 50–104
    d. 100–150

42. Most ear cleaning solutions have what property if the tympanic membrane is not intact?
    a. Ceruminolytic
    b. Antimicrobial
    c. Ototoxic
    d. Vestibulitis

43. When speaking with a client, when you ask for clarification, you are using what type of listening?
    a. Reflective
    b. Active
    c. Controlling
    d. Cheerful

44. What is the primary goal of nutritional assessment?
    a. To establish species normals
    b. To determine who is at risk for malnutrition
    c. To assess dehydration
    d. To determine normal growth rates

45. With what conditions can hyperthermia be associated?
    a. Malnutrition, vomiting
    b. Diarrhea, tenesmus
    c. Anemia, arrhythmias
    d. Infection, sepsis

46. Cats housed in catteries have a higher incidence of what type of diseases?
    a. FLUTD
    b. Upper respiratory
    c. Intestinal parasites
    d. Hyperthermia

47. How can the eyes be protected from exposure to soap when bathing an animal?
    a. Applying ophthalmic lubricating ointment
    b. Using an Elizabethan collar
    c. Cotton balls
    d. All shampoos are gentle, this is not a problem

48. At what position around the rectum are the anal glands found?
    a. 12 and 6
    b. 3 and 9
    c. 4 and 8
    d. 2 and 10

49. What needs to be considered when applying topical medications?
    a. The absorption rate of the medication
    b. Accidental oral ingestion should be prevented
    c. Twice as much needs to be used to account for poor absorption
    d. The color of the animal's coat

50. What is a reason for placement of an intravenous catheter?
    a. Administration of oral medications
    b. Management of hypothermia
    c. Prevent ototoxicity
    d. Fluid administration

39

CASE SCENARIO

You are helping Dr. Schwartz and Tammi, his technician, complete their records, and need to transcribe their patient notes into the hospital SOAP template.

Be sure to indicate which findings are abnormal or outside the normal reference range.

Jack Humbarger is a 3-year-old DSH, brown and black m/n cat. His presenting complaint is swelling of his left nictitan membrane, conjunctivitis, and clear ocular discharge. This has been worsening over the previous 5 days. His weight is 14# with a BCS of 4/5. Ears are clean and dry. His appetite is normal, and he is eating Pro Plan LiveClear dry. His temp is 102.5°F, HR 100 bpm, pulse matches HR, RR 20 bpm. His mucous membranes are pink and moist with a capillary refill time of <2 seconds. He was given 100 mg of gabapentin before today's visit.

On PE, all findings were within normal limits, coat is sleek and well groomed, except for his eye examination, and a clear nasal discharge is seen on his left nares. There is swelling on the OS conjunctiva and nictitans was elevated, as well as a large amount of clear ocular drainage. OD was normal. There is obvious squinting and discomfort noted OS, Glasgow pain scale 12/20.

Jack is up-to-date on all of his vaccines and is receiving monthly Revolution for heartworm prevention.

Diagnostics:
- Schirmer tear test: OD 15 mm, OS 30 mm
- Fluorescein staining: no stain uptake OU
- Intraocular pressure: 15 mm Hg OD, 18 mm Hg OS

Differentials:
- Herpes
- Mycoplasma
- Trauma

Treatment:
- Clean eyes well twice daily before medications.
- Tobramycin drops: 2 drops OS TID × 10 days
- Doxycycline capsules: 1 capsule opened and mixed with food BID × 10 days
- Buprenorphine: 2 mg (0.02 mL) PO BID × 3 days

Recheck:
Recheck eyes every 2 weeks. Contact us for a sooner recheck if any abnormal changes are noted.

Complete all gray sections in the SOAP form for this case.

Date: 01/01/01		
Patient name:		
Client name:		
Presenting complaint:		
	⬆⬇ Indicate if the findings are abnormal or normal	
Vitals:		
Temp:		
HR:		
RR:		
MM/CRT:		
Weight:		
BCS:		
Pre-visit pharmaceuticals:		
PE Findings:		Differentials:
General appearance		
MM		
Eyes		
Ears		
Nose		Diagnostic Plan:
Oral cavity		
Abdomen		

Date: 01/01/01		
Cardiovascular		
Respiratory		Treatment Plan:
Genitourinary		
Integument		
Musculoskeletal		Recheck:
Rectal		
Pain assessment		
Vaccines:		Record completed by:
RCP		
Rabies		
Heartworm Prevention		
Type		
Frequency		

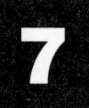

7 Anatomy and Physiology

LEARNING OBJECTIVES

After reviewing this chapter, the reader will be able to:

- Describe types of cells and tissues of the body.
- List the names of organs and structures that make up the various body systems.
- Describe the ways in which organs and body systems function and interact.
- Describe the general and special senses of the body and their functions.
- Differentiate between exocrine and endocrine glands.

FILL IN THE BLANK

1. The purpose of connective tissue is to _____ _____.

2. Adipose connective tissue consists of _____.

3. Loose connective tissues include _____ fibers, reticular fibers, and elastic fibers.

4. Elastic fibers provide some degree of _____.

5. Long bones have two parts: _____ and _____.

6. Flat bones provide maximum area for _____.

7. The largest sesamoid bone is the _____.

8. Most of the bones of a bird are _____ bones because they _____.

9. The surface at which a bone forms a joint with another bone is the _____.

10. A condyle is usually found on the _____.

11. A fossa is a _____, usually occupied by a muscle or tendon.

12. A lump or bump on the surface of a bone is called a _____.

13. The bones found in the neck region are the _____.

14. The thoracic vertebrae are found _____ _____.

15. The hind limb is termed the _____.

16. The thoracic limb is the _____.

17. The carpus is located between _____ and _____.

18. The purpose of the patella is to _____.

19. An example of a fibrous joint is _____.

20. Feathers and scales are part of the _____ in the nonmammalian species.

21. The largest organ in the body is the _____.

22. An albino animal has a total lack of _____.

23. Hair follicles, sebaceous glands, sudoriferous glands, and arrector pili muscles are found in the _____ of the skin.

24. The largest and main artery of the heart is the _____.

25. The primary function of the respiratory system is _____.

26. The upper fourth premolar and lower first molar in the dog are referred to as the _____teeth.

27. There are _____ pairs of cranial nerves.

28. The "fight-or-flight" reaction is produced by the _____ nervous system.

29. The "rest-and-restore" response is produced by the _____ nervous system.

30. The cat is an _____ ovulator.

LISTS

1. List the four basic tissues that make up the animal body:
   1. _____
      _____
   2. _____
      _____
   3. _____
      _____

4. _____

2. List the six types of connective tissue:

   1. _____

   2. _____

   3. _____

   4. _____

   5. _____

   6. _____

3. What are the three types of fibers found in loose connective tissue?

   1. _____

   2. _____

   3. _____

4. List the types of bones found in the mammal skeleton and give one example of each:

   1. _____

   2. _____

   3. _____

   4. _____

   5. _____

5. List the bones of the pelvic limb from proximal to distal:

   1. _____

   2. _____

   3. _____

4. _____

5. _____

6. _____

7. _____

8. _____

6. The axial skeleton comprises what four bones?

   1. _____

   2. _____

   3. _____

   4. _____

   5. _____

7. List the three pairs of bones that make up the pelvis in the adult animal:

   1. _____

   2. _____

   3. _____

8. List the three main types of joints and their movement:

   1. _____

   2. _____

   3. _____

9. Synovial joints allow for six potential joint movements. List them:

   1. _____

   2. _____

   3. _____

4. _____

   _____

5. _____

   _____

6. _____

   _____

10. List the three segments of the small intestine:

    1. _____

       _____

    2. _____

       _____

    3. _____

       _____

MULTIPLE CHOICE

1. Which type of muscle fibers are found in the pelvic limb?
   a. Smooth
   b. Rough
   c. Cardiac
   d. Skeletal

2. Which type of glands secrete directly into the bloodstream?
   a. Endocrine
   b. Lacrimal
   c. Sebaceous
   d. Goblet

3. What is the largest artery?
   a. Vena cava
   b. Carotid
   c. Aorta
   d. Ventricle

4. Which part of the circulatory system returns the blood to the heart?
   a. Arteries
   b. Veins
   c. Capillary
   d. Venules

5. Which vein carries nutrient-rich blood from the intestines to the liver?
   a. Aorta
   b. Vena cava
   c. Portal
   d. Cephalic

6. What is the basic unit of the nervous system?
   a. Fibron
   b. Neuron
   c. Venules
   d. Effector

7. In what organ is the olfactory sense located?
   a. Mouth
   b. Ear
   c. Nose
   d. Eyes

8. Equilibrium is what type of special sense?
   a. Mechanical
   b. Chemical
   c. Electromagnetic
   d. Thermal

9. Where do the epithelial tissues derive their nourishment?
   a. The vessels of the epithelium
   b. The dendrites and axons
   c. The underlying connective tissues
   d. The dermis

10. How many incisor teeth do cats and dogs have (counting both mandibular and maxillary teeth)?
    a. 8
    b. 10
    c. 12
    d. 14

11. What is the most common dental problem in dogs and cats older than 5 years?
    a. Stomatitis
    b. Periodontitis
    c. Enamel erosion
    d. Dental padding

12. Which part of the female reproductive tract "catches" the ova after the follicle has ruptured?
    a. infundibulum
    b. corpus luteum
    c. uterus
    d. cervix

13. What is the hardest material in the body?
    a. bone
    b. cartilage
    c. tooth enamel
    d. integument

14. What are the digits called in dogs and cats?
    a. metacarpals
    b. tarsus
    c. limbs
    d. phalanges

15. What type of joints do not allow any movement?
    a. Cartilaginous
    b. Fibrous
    c. Sesamoid
    d. Synovial

16. What type of tissue are claws and hooves composed of?
    a. keratinized
    b. erector
    c. hypodermis
    d. enamel

17. Sebaceous glands are responsible for production of what?
    a. saliva
    b. hydrochloric acid
    c. bile
    d. sebum

18. Under what tissues is a subcutaneous injection given?
    a. dermis
    b. epidermis
    c. hypodermis
    d. keratin

19. What is responsible for the color of hair?
    a. the shaft
    b. the root
    c. the erector pili muscle
    d. the melanocytes

20. When a dog's hackles stand up, what part of the hair is responsible?
    a. the shaft
    b. the root
    c. the erector pili muscle
    d. the melanocytes

21. What is the top portion of the heart?
    a. mitral valve
    b. atrium
    c. ventricle
    d. aorta

22. What heart valve is located between the right atrium and the right ventricle?
    a. tricuspid
    b. mitral
    c. pulmonary
    d. aortic

23. Which organ connects the placenta to the fetus?
    a. uterus
    b. cervix
    c. fallopian tube
    d. umbilical cord

24. What is another name for the larynx?
    a. nares
    b. voice box
    c. esophagus
    d. glottis

25. What can happen if an animal receives a gunshot wound to the chest?
    a. the lungs collapse
    b. the blood pressure increases
    c. the omentum covers over the hole
    d. the dog dies immediately from DIC

26. The functional unit for the kidneys is composed of what?
    a. cortex
    b. pelvis
    c. ureter
    d. nephron

27. Which part of the intestinal tract is responsible for the absorption of excess water?
    a. duodenum
    b. ileum
    c. jejunum
    d. colon

28. In which portion of the intestinal tract does the absorption of nutrients occur?
    a. duodenum
    b. ileum
    c. jejunum
    d. colon

29. What is the largest portion of the brain?
    a. cerebrum
    b. cerebellum
    c. brain stem
    d. pelvis

30. What muscles control the size of the pupil in the eye?
    a. erector pili
    b. triceps
    c. iris
    d. lacrimal

31. Which organ removes the liquid by-products from the body?
    a. intestinal tract
    b. liver
    c. lungs
    d. kidneys

32. What is the primary function of the reproductive tract in mammals?
    a. production of hormones
    b. maintenance of the species
    c. sympathetic movement
    d. asexual reproduction

33. What is the main purpose of the scrotum in male animals?
    a. regulate the temperature of the testes
    b. control ovulation
    c. production of sperm
    d. production of the sexual hormones

34. Where are sperm formed in an intact male dog?
    a. epididymis
    b. bulbourethral gland
    c. vas deferens
    d. seminiferous tubules

35. Who has mammary glands in mammals?
    a. males
    b. females
    c. males and females
    d. neither males nor females

36. Which lymphoid organ is responsible for "jump-starting" the immune system?
    a. thyroid
    b. spleen
    c. thymus
    d. lymph nodes

37. What structure transports urine from the renal pelvis to the bladder?
    a. ureter
    b. urethra
    c. vas deferens
    d. infundibulum

38. What is the longest cranial nerve?
    a. olfactory
    b. vagus
    c. optic
    d. patellar

39. Which gland is responsible for the production of tears?
    a. pancreas
    b. posterior pituitary
    c. thymus
    d. lacrimal

40. Which leukocytes are responsible for production of antibodies?
    a. neutrophils
    b. eosinophils
    c. monocytes
    d. lymphocytes

41. B-cell lymphocytes are responsible for production of specific antigens, what part of the immune system is this?
    a. humoral
    b. cellular
    c. killer B-cells
    d. acquired

42. The contraction phase of the cardiac cycle occurs during what?
    a. diastole
    b. intake
    c. systole
    d. atrium

43. What is the process of engulfing material in the bloodstream called?
    a. antigenic stimulation
    b. phagocytosis
    c. erythrogenesis
    d. activation

44. A patent ductus arteriosus is a congenital abnormality seen in which organ system?
    a. renal
    b. immune
    c. lungs
    d. cardiac

45. Transferring antibodies from the mother to the newborn is done through ingestion of what material?
    a. colostrum
    b. saliva
    c. sebum
    d. microbiome

46. What dome-shaped muscle separates the thoracic and abdominal cavities in mammals?
    a. intercostals
    b. capillary
    c. alveoli
    d. diaphragm

47. Where is the actual site of gas exchange in the lungs?
    a. alveoli
    b. venules
    c. arterioles
    d. bronchioles

48. The relaxation of the heart chambers happens during which phase?
    a. diastole
    b. intake
    c. systole
    d. atrium

49. Which protein is responsible for the red color in blood?
    a. albumin
    b. myofibrils
    c. hemoglobin
    d. axons

50. Which protein found in plasma is responsible for forming a blood clot?
    a. fibrin
    b. albumin
    c. globulin
    d. hemoglobin

Indicate the name of the appropriate bone on each numbered line. For the spine, provide the name for each section.

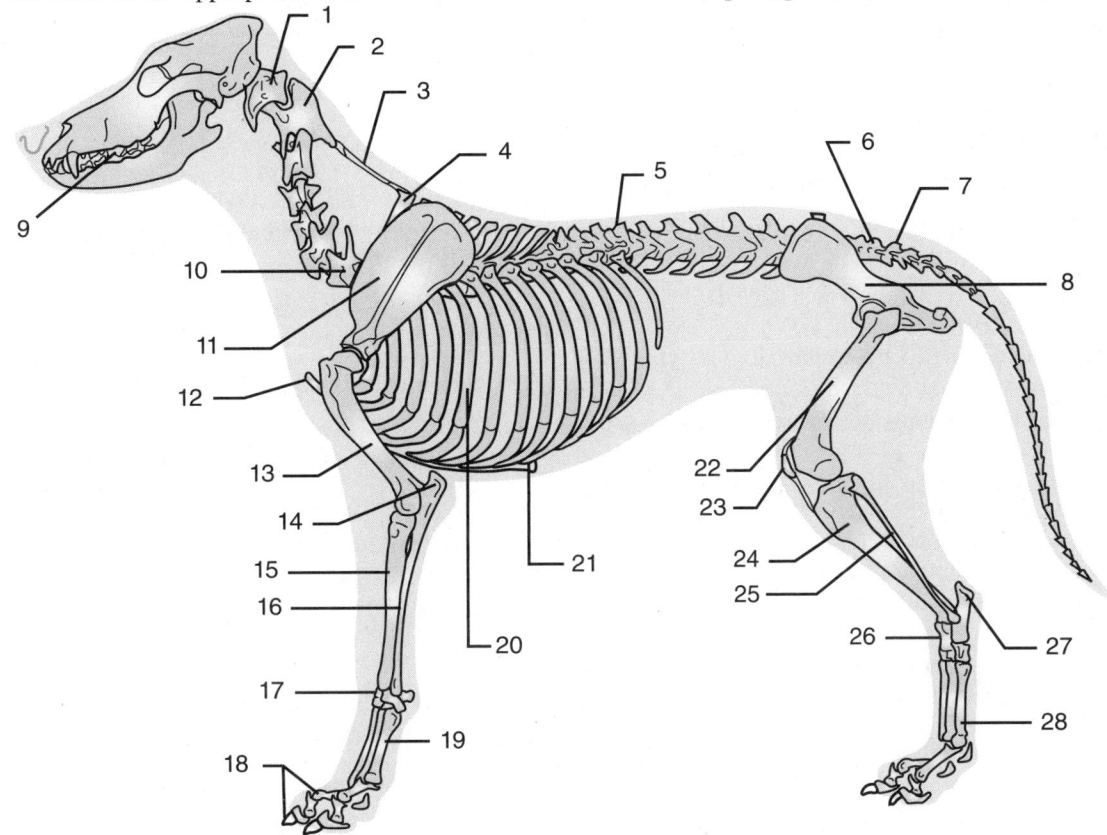

From Colville TP, Bassert JM: *Clinical anatomy and physiology for veterinary technicians*, ed 3, St. Louis, 2016, Elsevier.

1. _____

2. _____

3. _____

4. _____

5. _____

6. _____

7. _____

8. _____

9. _____

10. _____

11. _____

12. _____

13. _____

14. _____

15. _____

16. _____

17. _____

18. _____

19. _____

20. _____

21. _____

22. _____

23. _____

24. _____

25. _____

26. _____

27. _____

28. _____

8 Pharmacology and Pharmacy

FILL IN THE BLANK

1. An example of a drug that can be inactivated by violent shaking of the vial is _____.

2. Tuberculin and insulin syringes are available with attached _____ -gauge needles.

3. The larger the gauge number on a needle, the _____ the needle.

4. Needles larger than 1 inch are used for _____ and _____.

5. _____ medications may be supplied in single-dose vials, multidose vials, ampules, or large-volume bottles or bags.

6. For veterinarians to legally use, prescribe, or buy a controlled substance from an approved manufacturer or distributor, they must have obtained a _____ number from the DEA.

7. The ideal range of drug concentration that minimizes detrimental effects and maximizes benefits is referred to as the _____ range.

8. A drug's _____ is the amount of drug administered at one time.

9. The time between administration of separate drug doses is referred to as the _____.

10. Parenteral drugs are administered by _____.

11. Per os drugs are administered by _____.

12. Topically administered drugs are administered by _____ them to the skin.

13. Injection of a drug outside the blood vessel is an extravascular or _____ injection.

14. Intramuscular (IM) administration involves injecting the drug into a _____.

15. Subcutaneous (SC or SQ) injections are administered under the _____.

16. Intradermal (ID) injections are administered within the _____.

17. Intraperitoneal (IP) injections are administered into the _____.

18. Drugs or functions related to the stomach are called _____.

19. Drugs or functions related to the small intestine are referred to as _____.

20. Drugs and functions related to the colon are termed _____.

21. Drugs that are used to induce vomiting are referred to as _____.

22. Overuse of _____ drugs can produce Cushing syndrome.

23. To increase uterine contractions in animals with dystocia related to a weakened or fatigued uterus, the veterinarian commonly uses _____.

24. Drugs that kill or inhibit the growth of microorganisms or "microbes," such as bacteria, protozoa, viruses, or fungi, are called _____.

25. The ability to survive in the presence of antimicrobial drugs is referred to as drug _____.

26. The proprietary name of a drug is also referred to as its _____ name.

27. _____ are classified by generations, according to when they were first developed.

28. Compounds that kill various types of internal parasites are called _____.

29. _____ interferes with the development of the flea's chitin, which is essential for proper egg formation and development of the larval exoskeleton.

30. Drugs that relieve pain or discomfort by blocking or reducing the inflammatory process are called _____.

31. Cats are very sensitive to the OTC NSAID medication _____ and it is not generally recommended for clients to give.

32. Chemical agents that kill or prevent the growth of microorganisms on living tissues are called _____.

33. Chemical agents that kill or prevent the growth of microorganisms on inanimate objects are called _____.

34. A kilogram contains _____ grams and is abbreviated _____.

35. The abbreviation for the prefix micro- is _____ and refers to a unit that is a power of 10 of _____.

SHORT ANSWER

1. Describe the differences between a nonproprietary (generic) drug name and a proprietary (trademark) drug name.

   _____

   _____

2. Drug manufacturers and distributors are required to identify a controlled substance on its label with a capital C followed by a Roman numeral, which denotes the drug's theoretical potential for abuse. Define the potential for abuse and provide two examples of drugs for each drug classification:

   CI _____

   CII_____

   CIII _____

   CIV _____

   CV _____

3. List the components that the FDA states must be present on a drug container label.

   _____

   _____

   _____

   _____

   _____

   _____

   _____

   _____

DOSAGE CALCULATIONS

1. A 6-lb cat is prescribed amoxicillin at 5 mg/kg twice a day for 7 days. The oral medication has a concentration of 50 mg/mL. How many milliliters will the cat need per day?

2. A 30-lb cocker spaniel is to get a ketamine and diazepam induction IV, and the dose is 0.025 mL/lb for each. How much ketamine and diazepam will you draw up?

3. A 44-lb dog requires amoxicillin. The veterinarian prescribes 10 mg/kg, and the concentration is 100 mg/mL. How much amoxicillin will you give?

4. A 50-lb dog requires a carprofen dose of 2.2 mg/kg BID for 7 days. The drug is available in 25 mg, 75 mg, and 100 mg chewable tablets. What size tablet should be used, and how many tablets must be dispensed?

5. A litter of five puppies has been diagnosed with *Toxocara* spp. roundworms. The puppies weigh 3# each. Treatment is fenbendazole liquid 50 mg/kg q 24h x 3 days, mixed with food. The fenbendazole liquid has a concentration of 100 mg/mL. How much does each individual puppy get each day, and how much needs to be sent home to treat all five puppies for 3 days?

MULTIPLE CHOICE

1. Lactulose is commonly used as a laxative. What class of nutrient is it?
   a. Protein/amino acid
   b. Fat/lipid
   c. Carbohydrate/fiber
   d. Fat-soluble vitamin

2. Under what conditions should an antitussive be used?
   a. The animal has a productive cough
   b. The animal has a nonproductive cough
   c. The animal is vomiting
   d. The animal is dyspneic

3. What additional action is provided by the addition of sorbitol to activated charcoal?
   a. Cathartic
   b. Antitussive
   c. Antinausea
   d. Ileus

4. Which type of drugs can be given intravenously?
   a. Enteral
   b. Suppository
   c. Topical
   d. Parenteral

5. Antimicrobial drugs kill or inhibit the growth of what class of microorganisms?
   a. Bacteria and protozoa
   b. Virus and fungi
   c. Virus and bacteria
   d. Fungi, virus, bacteria, and protozoa

6. A vermicide is an anthelmintic that does what?
   a. Removes mites and lice from the environment
   b. Kills worms
   c. Paralyzes worms
   d. Inhibits parasitic molting

7. NSAIDs provide what action within the body?
   a. Relieve pain by blocking or reducing the inflammatory process
   b. Induce and maintain anesthesia
   c. Provide muscle relaxation and loss of consciousness
   d. A combination of two drugs that reduces CNS excitation

8. What must a cell have to be able to respond to a specific drug?
   a. An essential fatty acid
   b. Hormones
   c. Receptors
   d. Buffers

9. What is a drug that must be altered by the body to become effective called?
   a. Metabolite
   b. Toxin
   c. By-product
   d. Depolarizers

10. Which class of antibiotics are classified by generations?
    a. Penicillins
    b. Cephalosporins
    c. Aminoglycosides
    d. Fluoroquinolones

11. What is a medication that does not require a written prescription from a veterinarian called?
    a. Over-the-counter
    b. Nutraceuticals
    c. Therapeutic
    d. Scheduled

12. What is a surgical scrub designed to kill or prevent the growth of microorganisms on living tissue classified as?
    a. Bacteriostatic
    b. Antiseptic
    c. Disinfectant
    d. Sterilizer

13. Common bleach is classified as what type of disinfectant?
    a. Phenol
    b. Quaternary ammonium
    c. Alcohol
    d. Chlorine

14. Sanitizers that contain quaternary ammonium should not be used on what surfaces?
    a. High-touch surfaces
    b. Food bowls
    c. Floors
    d. Anesthetic equipment

15. What is a medication that helps to increase the fluidity of mucus in the respiratory tract called?
    a. Expectorant
    b. Antitussive
    c. NSAID
    d. Opioid

16. What is a drug that directly neutralizes acid molecules in the stomach or rumen called?
    a. Nonsystemic antacid
    b. Systemic antacid
    c. Antiulcer
    d. Motility modifier

17. What type of medication would be prescribed to an animal that has congestive heart failure and needs to have excess fluid accumulation removed through the kidneys?
    a. Vasodilator
    b. Positive inotrope
    c. Calcium channel blocker
    d. Diuretic

18. Aminophylline is useful under what conditions?
    a. Congestive heart failure
    b. Severe large bowel diarrhea
    c. Smooth muscle constriction in the lungs
    d. Thinning of the bile in the gall bladder

19. What condition is produced by an emetic in the gastrointestinal tract?
    a. Vomiting
    b. Ileus
    c. Absorbs toxins
    d. Antidiarrheal

20. Which drug is used to treat gastric ulcers by acting as a band-aid?
    a. Capromorelin
    b. Ranitidine
    c. Sucralfate
    d. Morphine

21. Which drug is a dissociated anesthetic?
    a. Thiopental
    b. Propofol
    c. Diazepam
    d. Ketamine

22. Butorphanol is in what class of drug?
    a. Analgesic
    b. NSAID
    c. Anesthetic
    d. Dissociative

23. Which class of drugs has antiinflammatory effects?
    a. Insulin
    b. Glucocorticoids
    c. Progesterones
    d. Opioids

24. Which drug is a glucocorticoid?
    a. Prednisolone
    b. Diazepam
    c. Ketamine
    d. Fentanyl

25. What process determines the route a drug is given?
    a. Distribution
    b. Manufacturing
    c. Pharmacokinetics
    d. Replication

26. What is the movement of drug molecules from the site of administration into the systemic circulation called?
    a. Biotransformation
    b. Absorption
    c. Metabolism
    d. Activation

27. Which drug is an example of a vasodilator?
    a. Propofol
    b. Aminophylline
    c. Furosemide
    d. Hydralazine

28. The dose of a drug refers to what amount?
    a. How much is administered at one time
    b. The time between each amount given
    c. The clearance time
    d. The route of administration

29. Which type of steroid hormones are produced by the adrenal cortex of animals?
    a. Glucocorticoids
    b. Testosterone
    c. Mineralocorticoid
    d. Thyroid

30. Which term refers to the ideal range of drug concentration?
    a. Dosage
    b. Therapeutic range
    c. Corticosterone index
    d. Biotransformation

31. What medications can be administered by mouth?
    a. Topical
    b. Rectal
    c. Parenteral
    d. Enteral

32. Flea and tick medications that are applied to the skin are examples of what type of administration?
    a. Topical
    b. Rectal
    c. Parenteral
    d. Enteral

33. Which antibiotic class can be associated with arthropathies (joint problems) in young animals?
    a. Fluoroquinolones
    b. Penicillins
    c. Cephalosporins
    d. Sulfonamides

34. A nonproprietary name of a drug can also be called what?
    a. Brand name
    b. Generic name
    c. Commercial name
    d. Therapeutic name

35. Which route of drug administration achieves the quickest effect?
    a. Topical
    b. PO
    c. IV
    d. IM

36. Loop diuretics can cause the loss of which mineral?
    a. Sodium
    b. Calcium
    c. Phosphorus
    d. Potassium

37. Which hormone disease is associated with an excessive glucocorticoid production?
    a. Cushing disease
    b. Addison disease
    c. Diabetes mellitus
    d. Hyperthyroidism

38. What is an abnormal electrical activity in the heart called?
a. Bradycardia
b. Tachycardia
c. Arrhythmia
d. Tachypnea

39. What is the dosage interval if a drug is to be administered q 12 hours?
a. SID
b. BID
c. TID
d. QID

40. What are the two main routes for drug elimination?
a. Enteral and parenteral
b. Digestion and absorption
c. Kidney and liver
d. Heart and lungs

41. What is a semisolid medication that can be inserted into the rectum for absorption across the intestinal wall?
a. Suppositories
b. Tincture
c. Enteric-coated tablet
d. Parenteral

42. Which term refers to an injection that is outside of the blood vessel?
a. Intravenous
b. Intra-arterial
c. Perivascular
d. Rectal

43. Maropitant citrate is an example of what type of drug?
a. Antibiotic
b. Anticonvulsant
c. Anthelmintic
d. Antiemetic

44. Which of these is an example of an inhalant anesthetic?
a. Isoflurane
b. Ketamine
c. Propofol
d. Alfaxalone

45. KBr (potassium bromide) is commonly combined with which medication to help control seizure activity?
a. Methocarbamol
b. Fentanyl
c. Acepromazine
d. Phenobarbital

46. Which type of injection is made directly into the abdominal cavity?
a. PO
b. IP
c. IM
d. ID

47. Which of these is a general term used to describe compounds that kill various types of internal parasites?
a. Antimicrobial
b. Antiseptic
c. Anthelmintic
d. Antibiotic

48. Which drug is an example of an internal antiparasitic?
a. Fenbendazole
b. Selamectin
c. Carbaryl
d. Permethrin

49. Which drug is an example of an NSAID?
a. Dexamethasone
b. Prednisone
c. Aspirin
d. Alcohol

50. Rescue is an example of what type of disinfectant?
a. Accelerated peroxide
b. Biguanide
c. Chlorine
d. Iodophor

CASE SCENARIO

Dr. Kennedy has asked you to reorganize the pharmacy. All the drugs have been pulled down and lined up on the counter. She has asked you to organize the drugs by their functions and then alphabetize them in each section.

The table below provides the proposed setup for the pharmacy shelves. Enter each drug by its generic name, alphabetically within the appropriate section. You will not be addressing the various drug concentrations.

You will also be organizing the locked box, where the scheduled drugs are kept. They will be organized by their schedule number and alphabetically within each section.

Antibiotics	Antifungals	Anthelmintic Internal	Antiparasitic External	Antiinflammatories
CII	**CIII**	**CIV**	**CV**	

Available medications:

Acetaminophen
Amitraz
Amoxicillin
Aspirin
Azithromycin
Buprenorphine
Carprofen
Cephalexin
Codeine
Dexamethasone SP
Diazepam
Doxycycline
Enrofloxacin
Fenbendazole
Gabapentin
Gentamicin
Griseofulvin
Imidacloprid
Itraconazole

Ivermectin
Ketamine
Ketoconazole
Melarsomine
Meloxicam
Methadone
Metronidazole
Morphine
Nitenpyram
Penicillin
Permethrin
Phenobarbital
Piperazine
Praziquantel
Prednisolone sodium succinate
Prednisone
Pyrantel
Selamectin
Sulfadiazine

LEARNING OBJECTIVES

After reviewing this chapter, the reader will be able to:

- Describe and explain surgical terminology.
- Discuss the principles of aseptic technique.
- Give examples of methods used to disinfect or sterilize surgical instruments and supplies.
- Describe procedures for preparing the surgical site and surgical team.
- Identify surgical instruments and explain their uses and maintenance.
- Compare and contrast types of suture needles and suture materials.
- Define the role of veterinary technicians in anesthesia and perioperative pain management.
- Describe the equipment used for anesthetizing animals.
- Prepare and maintain anesthetic machines and the associated equipment.
- List and describe the steps involved in anesthetizing animals for induction.
- Explain the procedures used in medicating and monitoring animals before, during, and after anesthesia.
- Prepare a small animal patient, anesthetic equipment, anesthetic agents, and accessories for general anesthesia.

SHORT ANSWER

1. After what length of time are skin sutures typically removed?

_____

_____

2. Other than sutures, what might be used for vessel ligation during surgery?

_____

_____

3. What is the most common form of gas sterilization found in the veterinary hospital, and for which equipment is it typically used?

_____

_____

_____

4. Name these scissors in order from left to right.

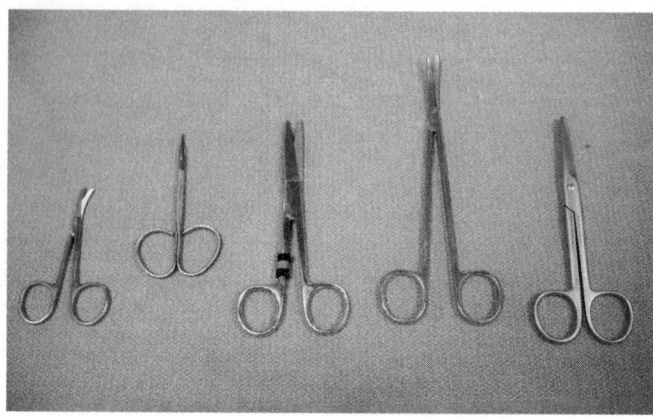

_____

_____

5. Why should hair be clipped liberally around the proposed surgical incision?

_____

_____

6. Explain the major function of surgical masks.

_____

_____

7. What is the purpose of daily monitoring of the body weight of a surgical patient?

_____

_____

8. Differentiate between contamination and infection of a wound.

_____

_____

9. Define pain.

_____

_____

MATCHING—SURGICAL INSTRUMENTS

Match the following surgical instruments with their primary function.

1. _____ Hemostatic forceps	A.	Used to incise tissue
2. _____ Needle holders	B.	Used for cutting tissue
3. _____ Retractors	C.	Grasp and manipulate curved needles
4. _____ Scissors	D.	Clamp and hold tissue and blood vessels
5. _____ Scalpels and blades	E.	Crushing instrument used to clamp blood vessels
6. _____ Tissue forceps	F.	Used to retract tissue and improve exposure

FILL IN THE BLANK

1. _____ is the term used to describe all precautions taken to prevent contamination or infection of a surgical wound.

2. Hospital-acquired infections are called _____.

3. Surgical mesh may be used to _____ or reinforce traumatized or devitalized tissues.

4. The unit used to create an environment of high-temperature, pressurized steam for sterilization of surgical instruments is called an _____.

5. _____ scissors have a blunt tip that, when introduced under the bandage edge, reduces the risk of cutting the underlying skin.

6. Organic nonabsorbable suture is available made of _____ or _____.

7. Surgical instrument manufacturers may recommend rinsing, cleaning, and sterilizing instruments in _____ because tap water contains minerals that cause discoloration and staining.

8. Subcutaneous infections frequently progress to _____.

9. Before sterilization, surgical drapes are folded so that the _____ can be properly positioned over the surgical site without contaminating the drape.

10. A _____ should be available to place needed supplies and equipment on the instrument table or Mayo stand in an operating room.

11. _____ needles have a sharp tip that pierces and spreads tissues without cutting them.

12. The _____ area is used for storage of surgical supplies.

13. It has been demonstrated that pain is more easily managed if analgesics are given _____ before a patient experiences pain.

14. Pain results from the stimulation of nerve endings called _____.

15. Procedures classified as "dirty" or nonsterile are usually performed in the _____ area.

16. When the sterility of an item is in question, always consider it _____.

17. The recommended method for verification of proper autoclave operation in veterinary clinics is _____.

18. A _____ is a monitoring device used to detect changes in oxygen saturation.

19. Before they are autoclaved, instruments with box locks and hinges should be lubricated with _____ or _____.

20. A _____ indicator is included in the middle of each pack to ensure that the inside of the pack is exposed to the appropriate sterilization temperatures.

SHORT ANSWER

1. What are five possible causes of wound dehiscence?

   1. _____
      _____
   2. _____
      _____
   3. _____
      _____
   4. _____
      _____
   5. _____
      _____

2. The four groups of nonabsorbable suture materials are:

1. _____

2. _____

3. _____

4. _____

3. List six pieces of surgical attire:

1. _____

2. _____

3. _____

4. _____

5. _____

6. _____

4. List at least three potential postoperative complications.

_____
_____
_____
_____
_____
_____
_____
_____
_____
_____

5. Describe what each of the following monitoring devices tells you about the patient.

Monitoring Device	Overview
Stethoscope	
Esophageal stethoscope	
Electrocardiograph	
Pulse oximeter	

Doppler ultrasound blood pressure	
Oscillometric blood pressure method	
Capnometer	

IDENTIFICATION

1. What gloving method is seen in the following figure? _____

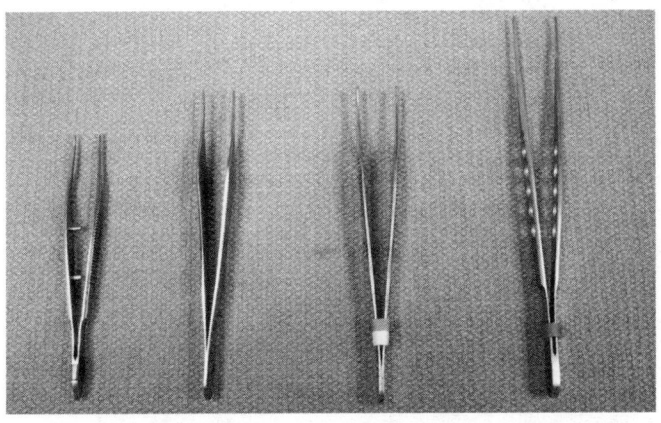

2. What procedure is pictured in the following figure? _____

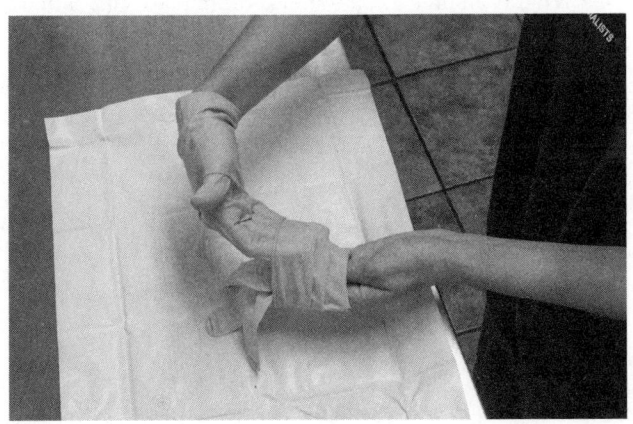

3. What sterilization equipment is seen in the following figure? _____

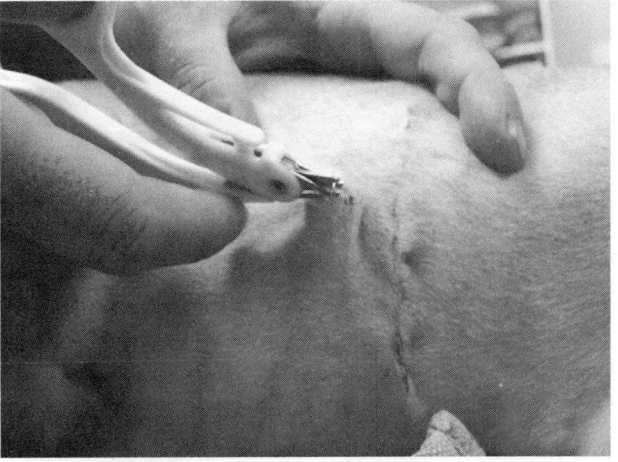

4. Examples of what type of suture are seen in the following figure? _____

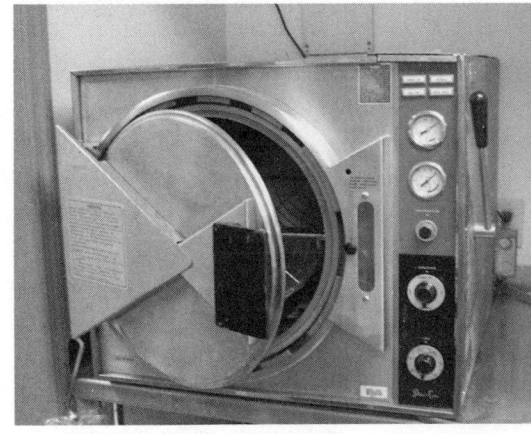

5. Identify both types of sterilization indicator tape seen in the following figure:

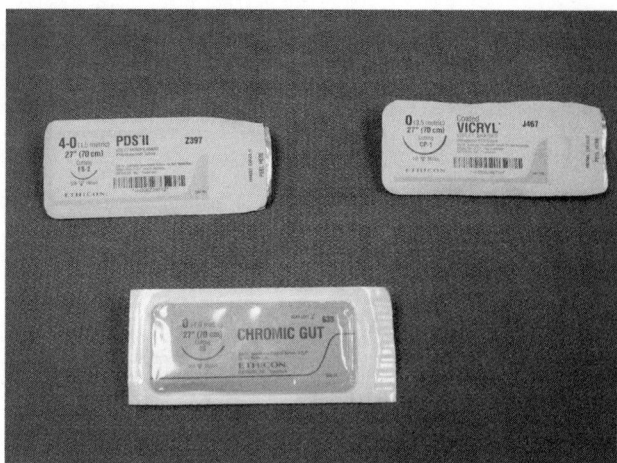

_____

_____

_____

6. What surgical instruments are pictured in the following figure?

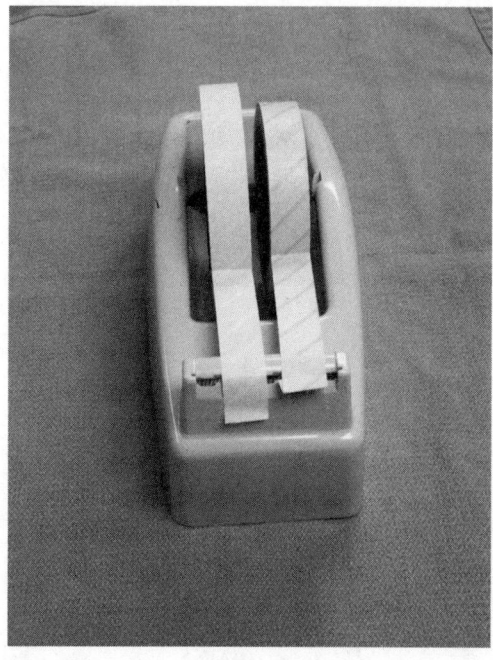

_____

7. What procedure is seen in the following figure? _____

_____

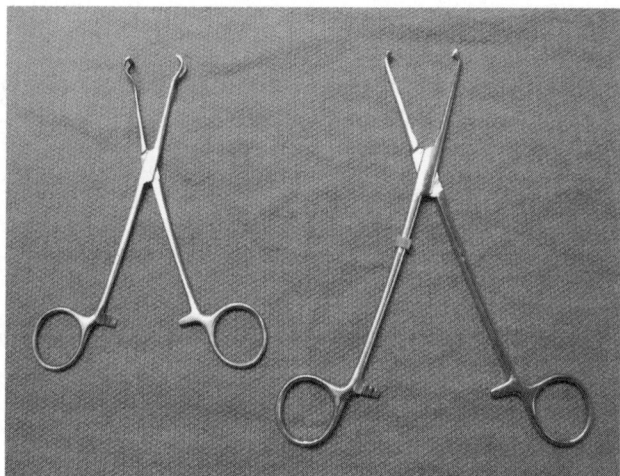

_____

MULTIPLE CHOICE

1. What is an infection in the abdominal cavity called?
   a. Encephalitis
   b. Peritonitis
   c. Dermatitis
   d. Osteomyelitis

2. What are instruments designed to cut or shape bone called?
   a. Osteotome
   b. Trephine
   c. Allis bone clamp
   d. Balfour retractor

3. When microorganisms in the body or wound multiply, this is called what?
   a. Aseptic technique
   b. Virulence
   c. Susceptibility
   d. Infection

4. What is an incision into the abdominal cavity called?
   a. Thoracotomy
   b. Hysterectomy
   c. Sternotomy
   d. Laparotomy

5. Which large crushing instruments are used to clamp blood vessels?
   a. Rat tooth forceps
   b. Blades
   c. Hemostats
   d. Retractors

6. What is an incision into the thoracic cavity called?
   a. Thoracotomy
   b. Hysterectomy
   c. Sternotomy
   d. Laparotomy

7. What is the destruction of most living pathogenic microorganisms on animate (living) objects called?
   a. Sterilization
   b. Disinfection
   c. Antiseptic
   d. Sporicidal

8. Which instrument is designed to bore holes into bone?
   a. Rongeur
   b. Osteotome
   c. Retractor
   d. Trephine

9. What is the primary objective of the surgeon and assistant performing a surgical scrub before gloving?
   a. To kill all of the surface pathogens
   b. Mechanical removal of dirt and reduction of the bacterial population
   c. To ensure that none of the bacterial pathogens on the patient are able to infect the surgical team
   d. So that no noxious fumes are produced during the surgical procedure

10. What is it called when the suture needle is joined to the suture?
    a. Swaged
    b. Frenched
    c. Eyed
    d. Threaded

11. What is an incision into the urethra called?
    a. Celiotomy
    b. Penectomy
    c. Urethrotomy
    d. Cystotomy

12. Which type of scissors are appropriate for use in cutting heavy tissue, such as fascia?
    a. Iris
    b. Mayo
    c. Metzenbaum
    d. Suture

13. Which piece of sterilization equipment creates high-temperature pressurized steam?
    a. Autoclave
    b. Cold sterile
    c. Ethylene oxide
    d. Biologic

14. What is a material called that is used to ligate blood vessels?
    a. Hemostat
    b. Suture
    c. Retractor
    d. Scissors

15. The use of a cauterizing needle tip generating heat in tissue with a high-frequency current, is called what?
    a. Electrocoagulation
    b. Electrocution
    c. Electrocautery
    d. Electrostimulation

16. Which of these is a self-retaining retractor with a set screw to maintain tension on tissues?
    a. Senn
    b. Balfour
    c. Gelpi
    d. Army-Navy

17. What is an incision into the intestines to remove a foreign body called?
    a. Laparotomy
    b. Enterotomy
    c. Gastrostomy
    d. Urethrostomy

18. Which tissue scissors are most appropriate for fine, thin tissue?
    a. Mayo
    b. Iris
    c. Metzenbaum
    d. Tenotomy

19. What is the surgical removal of the mammary glands called?
    a. Mastectomy
    b. Ovariohysterectomy
    c. Onychectomy
    d. Enterotomy

20. Which of these is a self-retaining retractor with a box lock to maintain tension on tissues?
    a. Senn
    b. Army-Navy
    c. Finochietto
    d. Gelpi

21. Which type of incision is performed when an animal is in lateral or standing?
    a. Ventral midline
    b. Paramedian
    c. Flank
    d. Paracostal

22. What can happen to the tissue when the muscle and skin sutures at an incision site break down?
    a. Herniation
    b. Evisceration
    c. Infection
    d. Abscess

23. What is pain management that is administered before a procedure called?
    a. Experimental
    b. Postoperative
    c. Preemptive
    d. Windup

24. Which piece of monitoring equipment is used to measure end-tidal CO_2?
    a. Pulse oximeter
    b. Esophageal stethoscope
    c. ECG
    d. Capnometer

25. Where, in relation to the circuit, is the vaporizer typically located for anesthetic gasses?
    a. Inside
    b. Outside
    c. Even
    d. Above

26. Which of these is a normal pulse oximetry reading?
    a. 35–45 mm Hg
    b. 120 mm Hg
    c. 95%–100%
    d. 120–150 bpm

27. What is defined as an unpleasant sensory or emotional experience associated with actual or potential tissue damage?
    a. Dehiscence
    b. Inflammation
    c. Nociception
    d. Pain

28. Which common antimicrobial agent works to mechanically remove microorganisms?
    a. Soap
    b. Quaternary ammonium compounds
    c. Biguanide compounds
    d. Phenols

29. Which common disinfectant is not effective against viruses?
    a. Glutaraldehyde
    b. Iodophors
    c. Alcohol, iodine combination
    d. Quaternary ammonium

30. Which term describes any disturbance of the heart's rhythm resulting in fewer-than-normal heartbeats?
    a. Tachycardia
    b. Arrhythmia
    c. Dyspnea
    d. Mitral regurgitation

31. What is the top pressure that should be achieved when bagging or providing positive pressure ventilation for an animal under anesthesia?
    a. 5–10 mm Hg
    b. 15–20 cm H_2O
    c. 35–45 kg
    d. 95%–100%

32. How is carbon dioxide (CO_2) removed from an anesthetic circuit?
    a. Soda lime
    b. Scavenger
    c. Pop-off valve
    d. Through the blood

33. Which type of ultrasound device can a technician use to sense the presence or absence of flow in blood vessels?
    a. Capnometer
    b. Pulse oximeter
    c. Doppler
    d. ECG

34. Which kind of stethoscope can be placed during anesthesia at the level of the heart to amplify the heartbeat so that it is audible from a distance?
    a. Esophageal
    b. Rectal
    c. Pediatric bell
    d. None, there is not enough room for this use

35. What term describes elevated carbon dioxide levels in the blood?
    a. Tachycardia
    b. Tidal volume
    c. Hypercarbia
    d. Nonrebreathing

36. What part of an anesthetic machine determines the amount of oxygen that the animal receives?
    a. Pressure regulator valve
    b. Flowmeter
    c. Vaporizer
    d. Scavengers

37. What agents can be used to suppress the physiologic pain mechanisms that remain active during anesthesia?
    a. Analgesics
    b. Sedatives
    c. Anxiolytics
    d. Local blocks

38. What medical instrument can be used to obtain a view of the vocal folds and the glottis?
    a. Stethoscope
    b. Cystoscope
    c. Laryngoscope
    d. Laparoscopy

60

39. Which type of needle holders have a ratchet lock just distal to the thumb?
    a. Mayo-Hegar
    b. Mathieu
    c. Castroviejo
    d. Allis

40. Which type of suture needle allows suture to be threaded onto the needle?
    a. Swagged
    b. Keith
    c. Eyed
    d. Holeless

41. Which type of needles are used most commonly to close skin incisions?
    a. Taper
    b. Cutting
    c. Straight
    d. Side-cutting

42. How long does it typically take for absorbable sutures to lose most of their tensile strength?
    a. 10–14 days
    b. 2–3 weeks
    c. 4–6 weeks
    d. 60–90 days

43. Which type of organic nonabsorbable suture is preferred for cardiovascular surgeries?
    a. Silk
    b. Cotton
    c. Metal
    d. Chromic gut

44. What is the surgical removal of the testicles called?
    a. Onychectomy
    b. Hysterectomy
    c. Ostectomy
    d. Orchiectomy

45. What procedure can be done to save the fetuses when there is dystocia during labor?
    a. Cystotomy
    b. Hysterectomy
    c. Cesarean section
    d. CPR

46. Which type of retractor is double ended?
    a. Weitlaner
    b. Gelpi
    c. Finochietto
    d. Senn

47. Which of these tissue forceps have small serrations on the tips that cause minimal trauma but hold tissue securely?
    a. Brown-Adson
    b. Allis
    c. Mosquito
    d. Crile

48. Which type of small hemostatic forceps have transverse jaw serrations and are used to clamp small blood vessels?
    a. Kelly
    b. Carmalt
    c. Angiotribe
    d. Mosquito

49. Which type of large crushing forceps can be used to control large tissue bundles?
    a. Kelly
    b. Rochester-Carmalt
    c. Angiotribe
    d. Crile

50. This is a surgical procedure typically done to fix the stomach to the abdominal wall that decreases the risk of gastric torsion.
    a. Gastrectomy
    b. Gastrotomy
    c. Gastropexy
    d. Anastomosis

CASE SCENARIO

1. Go to https://www.cliniciansbrief.com/article/basic-surgery-kit. Identify the individual instruments found in the image "The Basic Surgery Kit." Start your identification at the upper left side and work across. Since you cannot see the serrations inside of the hemostats, indicate whether they are curved or straight and if they are mosquito hemostats.

   _____

   _____

   _____

2. The doctor wants 1 pack of nonabsorbable synthetic sutures and 1 pack of absorbable sutures for their pack. What suture material do you select?

   A. Nonabsorbable suture_____

   B. Absorbable suture _____

3. The first animal set for surgery today is a 5-year-old 50# Basset Hound named Dolly. She is having a spay. Please provide what organs are being removed.

   _____

   _____

   _____

10 Laboratory Procedures

LEARNING OBJECTIVES

After reviewing this chapter, the reader will be able to:

- Describe methods used to collect samples for laboratory examination.
- Describe the preparation of diagnostic samples for laboratory examination.
- List and describe common procedures used for hematologic examinations.
- List and describe methods for evaluation of hemostasis in dogs and cats.
- List and describe equipment needed for clinical chemistry and serology testing.
- List and describe the types of tests used in clinical chemistry testing.
- List the biochemical assays commonly performed to assess liver, kidney, and pancreatic function.
- List the types of immunologic tests and describe the test principles used in those tests.
- Discuss methods used to verify the accuracy of laboratory test results.
- List and describe methods used to collect samples of body tissues and fluids for laboratory examination.
- List and describe microbiologic tests commonly performed to identify bacterial and fungal pathogens.
- List tests commonly performed in analyzing urine specimens.
- List common internal parasites of dogs and cats.
- List common external parasites of dogs and cats.

MATCHING—TERMS

1. _____ Photosensitive reagent	A. Icterus
2. _____ Coombs test	B. Rapid immunomigration
3. _____ Study of microbes	C. Microbiology
4. _____ Immunochromatography	D. Packed cell volume
5. _____ Bacilli	E. Mycology
6. _____ Cocci	F. Chromogen
7. _____ Microhematocrit	G. Rising antibody titer
8. _____ Jaundice	H. Round-shaped bacteria
9. _____ Study of fungi	I. Rod-shaped bacteria
10. _____ Indicates active infection	J. Detects autoantibodies

MATCHING—MICROBIOLOGY

1. _____ Fungi	A. Broth media
2. _____ Multiple media in a single plate	B. Bullseye
3. _____ Thioglycolate	C. Dermatophyte test media
4. _____ Mueller-Hinton	D. Culture and sensitivity

SHORT ANSWER AND FILL IN THE BLANK

1. How would you prepare a 1:10 dilution of a patient sample?

   _____

   _____

   _____

2. Identify the organs/tissues with which these tests are associated:

   AST _____

   ALT _____

   ALP _____

   BUN _____

3. List at least four tests used to evaluate the pancreas:

   1. _____

   2. _____

   3. _____

   4. _____

4. Name the type of immunologic test that is most commonly used in veterinary practice.

   _____

5. How should samples from animals with suspected zoonoses be submitted?

   _____

   _____

6. Name the two most common uses of agglutination tests in small animal veterinary practice:

   _____

   _____

7. Of impression and scraping, which sample collection technique yields more cells?

   _____

   _____

8. The PCV is also known as the_____

   _____

9. List four methods of urine collection:

   1. _____

   2. _____

   3. _____

10. Gross examination of urine should include evaluation of color, _____, ___ _____, and _____.

11. List the four components of the complete urinalysis:

    1. _____

       _____

    2. _____

       _____

    3. _____

       _____

    4. _____

       _____

12. _____ is the preferred anticoagulant for hematology testing in mammals.

13. Parasites residing on the surface of the host are called _____

    _____.

14. Name the two main classifications of ticks:

    1. _____

       _____

    2. _____

       _____

15. Name the two main classifications of mites:

    1. _____

       _____

    2. _____

       _____

MULTIPLE CHOICE

1. What solution should be mixed with the feces when doing a fecal smear?
   a. saline
   b. distilled water
   c. lactated Ringer solution
   d. zinc sulfate

2. When should the fecal samples be examined?
   a. immediately after collection
   b. within 24 hours
   c. after a 72-hour incubation
   d. within 7 days

3. Which of these are examples of kidney function tests?
   a. AST and ALT
   b. fructosamine and glucose
   c. amylase and lipase
   d. BUN and creatinine

4. What is red-tinged plasma referred to as?
   a. hemolyzed
   b. icteric
   c. lipemic
   d. normal

5. What is yellow-tinged plasma referred to as?
   a. hemolyzed
   b. icteric
   c. lipemic
   d. normal

6. Why is it important to keep the sink and centrifuge separated from the laboratory equipment and microscope?
   a. to ensure you have a large enough working triangle
   b. to increase the size of the laboratory space
   c. to prevent accidental damage
   d. because state law requires a minimum of 5' between pieces of equipment

7. Which federal administration mandates specific laboratory practices that must be incorporated into the laboratory safety policy for each hospital?
   a. FDA
   b. USDA
   c. AVMA
   d. OSHA

8. When writing the results for a dilution performed in the laboratory, if the dilution was 1:5, and the results were 20, what would the final corrected results be?
   a. 5
   b. 25
   c. 100
   d. 150

9. Which type of microscope is found most commonly in veterinary hospitals?
   a. monocular
   b. binocular
   c. tungsten
   d. simple light

10. Routine, daily cleaning of a microscope can be done using what?
    a. 70% alcohol
    b. lens tissue paper
    c. fiber-free gauze squares
    d. hydrogen peroxide

11. What is the primary purpose of a centrifuge?
    a. incubate bacterial cultures
    b. determine urine specific gravity
    c. ensure safety measures are being followed
    d. separate substances of different densities

12. When using a microhematocrit centrifuge, what type of tubes are used?
    a. capillary tubes
    b. high-capacity conical tubes
    c. small-capacity blood tubes
    d. they accept any sized tube

13. What solutions can be measured by using a refractometer?
    a. plasma and urine
    b. whole blood and serum
    c. thinned fecal smears and urine
    d. skin scrapings and ear cytology

14. What solution is used to calibrate the refractometer?
    a. 0.9% saline
    b. distilled water
    c. 70% alcohol
    d. hydrogen peroxide

15. When using liquid chemistry reagents, what method can be used to decrease your exposure to potentially hazardous reagents?
    a. using unitized reagents
    b. allowing the liquid to dry out before use
    c. wearing chemo-protective gloves and a N95 mask
    d. configure the electrodes to use less reagent

16. Why are adaptations needed to human use hematology analyzers for use in veterinary patients?
    a. no adaptations are needed, the same equipment can be used
    b. there is variation in blood cell sizes in different animal species
    c. Veterinarians cannot spend the same amount of money on the equipment
    d. Veterinary patient hair can interfere with the machinery and special filters are required

17. Why is it recommended to still do a manual cell differential, even when an automated CBC has been done?
    a. to optimize the use of technician time
    b. because of inherent inaccuracies in cell line identification in all machines
    c. numerous morphologic abnormalities can be present and may not be identified by the machine
    d. naturally occurring platelet clumps can negatively affect the machine's ability to calculate the RBC indices

18. What temperature does an in-house incubator need to be able to maintain?
    a. 72°F/22°C
    b. 98°F/37°C
    c. 104°F/40°C
    d. 212°F/100°C

19. When using an incubator, what is the purpose of placing a small plate of water inside?
    a. it provides a negative control
    b. it helps to modulate the temperature
    c. it helps to maintain the proper humidity
    d. it automatically cleans up any bacterial residue inside

20. What is the recommended amount an animal should be fasted before blood collection?
    a. fasting is not required
    b. 60 minutes
    c. 4 hours
    d. 12 hours

21. What is the preferred site of collection when larger volumes of blood are required?
    a. cephalic vein
    b. femoral artery
    c. jugular vein
    d. carotid artery

22. What is the preferred anticoagulant for hematology testing in dogs and cats?
    a. lithium heparin
    b. EDTA
    c. sodium citrate
    d. no anticoagulant is required

23. Which anticoagulant is preferred for coagulation tests?
    a. lithium heparin
    b. EDTA
    c. sodium citrate
    d. no anticoagulant is required

24. RBC indices can provide information on what type of disease?
    a. intestinal parasite infections
    b. liver function
    c. renal function
    d. anemia

25. What type of equipment can be used for long-term storage of fluid samples?
    a. crisper drawer in a standard refrigerator
    b. upper, back corner of the refrigerator, inside a labeled box
    c. non–self-defrosting chest freezer
    d. upright self-defrosting freezer

26. What would be the color of an icteric plasma sample?
    a. straw
    b. red
    c. clear
    d. yellow

27. What can cause a lipemic sample?
    a. inadequate fasting
    b. using too small of a needle for blood collection
    c. a high-fiber diet
    d. this is normal for some species

28. A plasma sample that is tinged red is consistent with what problem?
    a. icterus
    b. lipemia
    c. hemolysis
    d. this is normal in adult animals

29. Which enzymes are associated with liver function?
    a. total protein and RBC count
    b. ALP and ALT
    c. lipase and amylase
    d. BUN and glucose

30. What protein is present in plasma samples but absent in serum samples?
    a. fibrinogen
    b. immunoglobulins
    c. total proteins
    d. albumin

31. With dehydration what changes can be seen in the total protein level?
    a. a decrease in albumin, but a normal globulin
    b. a decrease
    c. an elevation
    d. an increase in globulin with a normal albumin

32. Azotemia can be seen with increases in which chemistry value?
    a. AST
    b. bilirubin
    c. amylase
    d. BUN

33. What test can be done to determine the presence of specific disease-causing bacteria?
    a. centrifuged fecal sedimentation
    b. total protein using a refractometer
    c. culturing in an incubator
    d. urinalysis

34. What is the role of aseptic technique when collecting a sample that will be cultured?
    a. it helps prevent outside contamination of the sample
    b. it makes staining easier
    c. it ensures that the sample is kept at the correct temperature
    d. it separates the desired sample from normal flora

35. Exposure of prepared slides to formalin fumes is an example of what type of problem?
    a. aseptic technique
    b. cross contamination
    c. fungal exposure
    d. dilution

36. When doing screening cultures for bacterial, viral, and fungal infections, how many different samples need to be collected?
    a. 1 universal media sample
    b. 2, 1 for viral and 1 for bacterial and fungal
    c. 3, 1 for each type of sample being tested
    d. 4, 2 for bacterial and 1 each for viral and fungal

37. When should the sample be collected when testing for the presence of bacteria through culturing?
    a. before any treatment or antibiotics have been given
    b. within 12 hours of fluid therapy and antibiotic use
    c. within 24 hours of antibiotic use
    d. timing is not important if the bacteria are there, testing can be done at any time

38. For a dilute cytology sample, what can be done to concentrate the cells?
    a. evaporation in the incubator for 12 hours
    b. centrifugation
    c. mix with distilled water
    d. concentration with hydrogen peroxide

39. What type of tissue sample can be prepared from active lesions or surgical samples?
    a. histology
    b. swab
    c. impression
    d. fine needle aspirate

40. Which type of cytology collection uses a site preparation similar to venipuncture?
    a. impression
    b. cytology
    c. roll prep
    d. fine needle aspirate

41. What type of cells are associated with an inflammatory sample?
    a. erythrocytes
    b. neutrophils
    c. squamous epithelial
    d. basophils

42. Concerning histology, formalin is what type of material?
    a. stains acidic organelles
    b. stains basic organelles
    c. fixative
    d. clarifying agent

43. What needs to be done first when preparing to perform a urinalysis on a refrigerated sample?
    a. an adequate volume of fixative needs to be mixed with the sample
    b. centrifugation at the highest speed possible
    c. decanting into a sterile container
    d. bring it to room temperature

44. What sample collection technique is used for vaginal cytology?
    a. impression smear
    b. histology
    c. swab
    d. fine needle aspirate

45. When doing a urinalysis, chemical evaluation is done using what equipment?
    a. dipstick
    b. refractometer
    c. centrifuge
    d. hematology analyzer

46. An organism that lives inside another organism and derives its nourishment from them is called what?
    a. commensal
    b. opportunistic
    c. parasite
    d. definitive host

47. Roundworms, hookworms, and heartworms are all classified as what type of parasites?
    a. cestodes
    b. trematodes
    c. nematodes
    d. protozoans

48. Which intestinal parasite can be transmitted from the *Ctenocephalides* spp. flea to dogs and cats?
    a. *Dipylidium*
    b. *Dirofilaria*
    c. *Dioctophyma*
    d. *Diphyllobothrium*

49. *Demodex* spp. are classified as what type of parasites?
    a. mites
    b. flies
    c. ticks
    d. fleas

50. The zoonotic parasite, *Toxocara* spp. causes what disease in humans?
    a. toxoplasmosis
    b. hydatidosis
    c. visceral larva migrans
    d. giardiasis

CASE SCENARIO

You arrive at the clinic for your morning shift and want to get started on the preanesthetic needed for the animals who were admitted last night for surgery today.

Describe what samples are needed for each of these animals and what information these samples will provide the veterinarian.

1. **Duke** is an 18-month-old Bichon Frise who is in for an orchiectomy and deciduous teeth removal of 104, 204, 304, and 404. The doctor has requested an automated CBC with manual differential, a preanesthetic chemistry panel in-house (includes BUN, creatinine, AST, ALP, glucose, and total protein), heartworm testing using whole blood on an ICT test, fecal floatation via centrifugation, and urinalysis.

A. CBC, sample needed: _____

_____

_____

B. CBC, information provided: _____

_____

_____

C. Manual differential, sample needed: _____

_____

_____

D. Manual differential, information provided: _____

_____

_____

E. Chemistry, sample needed: _____

_____

_____

F. Chemistry, information provided (provide organ system that is evaluated):

1) BUN _____

_____

2) Creatinine _____

_____

3) AST _____

_____

4) ALP _____

_____

5) Glucose_____

6) Total protein _____

_____

G. Heartworm, sample required: _____

_____

_____

H. Heartworm, information provided: _____

_____

_____

I. Fecal, sample needed: _____

_____

_____

J. Fecal, information provided: _____

_____

_____

K. Urinalysis, sample needed: _____

_____

_____

L. Urinalysis, materials needed:

1) Specific gravity _____

2) Presence of glucose _____

3) Presence of formed elements _____

2. **Sylvester** is a 6-month-old female DSH who is in for her OHE. She was found by her owners at a neighbor's barn and has not been tested for feline leukemia (FeLV) or feline immunodeficiency virus (FIV). She also has a unilateral (OS) green ocular discharge. The doctor wants a swab cytology from the conjunctival sac to be sent to your reference lab looking for mycoplasma and herpes virus. While you are doing your preliminary examination, you note a crusty, dry brown discharge in both ears. You decide to collect cytology looking for ear mites. The doctor has requested an automated CBC with manual differential, a preanesthetic chemistry panel in-house (includes BUN, creatinine, AST, ALP, glucose, and total protein), FeLV/FIV testing using whole blood and an ELISA test, and fecal floatation via centrifugation.

Since we already know what information the CBC, manual diff, preanesthetic chemistry panel, and fecal can tell us, please answer these questions about Sylvester and her tests.

A. FeLV/FIV testing, sample required: _____

_____

_____

B. FeLV/FIV testing, what does the chromogen bind to in this test? _____

_____

_____

_____

C. Ocular cytology, sample required: _____

_____

_____

_____

D. Ocular cytology, transport requirements: _____

_____

_____

_____

E. Ear cytology, sample required: _____

_____

_____

F. Ear cytology, are these burrowing or nonburrowing mites? _____

_____

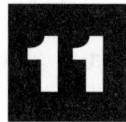# Diagnostic Imaging

LEARNING OBJECTIVES

After reviewing this chapter, the reader will be able to:

- Describe the components of the x-ray machine and the function of each part.
- Explain how x-rays are produced.
- Discuss the factors that affect radiographic quality.
- Describe techniques and devices used to optimize radiographic quality.
- Discuss the dangers of radiation and methods to avoid radiation injury.
- Describe the procedures used to develop radiographs.
- Explain the proper positioning of animals for various radiographic studies.
- Describe the basic physics of ultrasound.
- List the components of ultrasound machines and the function of each part.
- List the non–x-ray imaging modalities and provide an overview of each.

FILL IN THE BLANK

1. Denser tissues, such as bone, absorb greater amounts of x-rays and appear _____ _____.

2. The National Council on Radiation Protection and Measurements recommends that the dose for occupationally exposed persons not exceed _____ per year.

3. The MPD for nonoccupational persons is _____% of the dose for occupationally exposed persons, or _____ per year.

4. What does ALARA stand for?_____ _____ _____

5. How long should the patient be fasted for GI endoscopy? _____ _____

6. Who is required to wear lead shielding when taking radiographs? _____ _____ _____

7. What does "rem" stand for? _____ _____ _____

8. A sievert equals how many rem? _____ _____ _____

9. What precautions should a pregnant person occupationally exposed to radiation take?_____ _____

10. What does a rad measure? _____ _____ _____

COMPLETE THE CHART

Body Part	Cranial or Proximal Landmark	Caudal or Distal Landmark	Center Landmark	Comments
Abdomen				Take at peak _____
Thorax				Take at peak _____
Pelvis			X	X
Stifle				X
Radius and ulna				X
Lumbar vertebrae			X	To increase detail _____

MATCHING—KEY TERMS

A. Terms Associated With Radiographic Quality

1. _____ Anode heel effect	A. Loss of detail resulting from geometric lack of sharpness
2. _____ Radiographic density	B. Unwanted density in the form of blemishes
3. _____ Radiographic contrast	C. Sharp interfaces between tissues and organs
4. _____ Subject density	D. Unequal distribution of the x-ray beam intensity
5. _____ Radiographic detail	E. Differences in radiographic density between adjacent areas on a radiographic image
6. _____ Artifacts	F. Degree of blackness on a radiograph
7. _____ Penumbra	G. Ability of the different tissue densities to absorb x-rays

B. Terms Associated With Positioning

1. _____ Ventral (V):	A. Situated closer to the point of attachment or origin
2. _____ Dorsal (D):	B. Situated on the caudal aspect of the rear limb, distal to the tarsus
3. _____ Medial (M):	C. Areas on the head situated toward the nose
4. _____ Lateral (L):	D. Body area situated toward the median plane or midline
5. _____ Cranial (Cr):	E. Situated away from the point of attachment or origin
6. _____ Caudal (Cd):	F. Structures or areas situated toward the head
7. _____ Rostral (R):	G. Body area situated toward the underside of quadrupeds
8. _____ Palmar (Pa):	H. Structures or areas situated toward the tail
9. _____ Plantar (Pl):	I. Situated on the caudal aspect of the front limb, distal to the carpus
10. _____ Proximal (Pr):	J. Body area situated toward the back or topline of quadrupeds
11. _____ Distal (Di):	K. Body area situated away from the median plane or midline

MULTIPLE CHOICE

1. Unequal distribution of the x-ray beam results in the phenomenon referred to as:
   a. penumbra effect
   b. heel effect
   c. ALARA
   d. hyperechoic

2. Which of the following choices is ordered from lowest subject density to greatest subject density?
   a. metal, bone, water, fat, and gas
   b. fat, water, gas, bone, and metal
   c. water, gas, fat, bone, and metal
   d. gas, fat, water, bone, and metal

3. Where should the radiation monitoring badge be worn?
   a. on your glove edge
   b. at your waist inside the gown
   c. at your collar outside the gown
   d. on the pocket of your scrub pants under the gown

4. Scatter will be more noticeable if there is a thicker patient and:
   a. lower kVp and larger field size
   b. lower kVp and smaller field size
   c. higher kVp and smaller field size
   d. higher kVp and larger field size

5. Which imaging modality would be used to visualize the structure and function of organs?
   a. radiographs
   b. MRI
   c. CT
   d. endoscopy

6. Collimation can be used to decrease what effect?
   a. penumbra
   b. heel
   c. patient motion
   d. intensifying

7. Under what conditions foreshortening of a limb can be seen?
   a. there is motion
   b. inadequate collimation has been done
   c. the leg is not parallel to the screen surface
   d. the contrast dye has been injected too slowly

8. If a film has been adequately collimated, what should be seen on the completed image?
   a. a white line all around
   b. a black line all around
   c. an image right up to the edge
   d. pixelation

9. If there was no image on a film that was exposed to radiation and it was processed normally, the film would appear what color?
   a. white
   b. blue
   c. green
   d. black

10. Which of these imaging modalities is *not* digital?
    a. Rare earth
    b. CR
    c. CCR
    d. DR

11. When producing digital images, how is the image seen?
    a. on radiographic film
    b. on a computer screen
    c. on special televisions
    d. on a view box

12. What is DICOM used for?
    a. production of radiation
    b. removing scatter radiation
    c. storage of digital images
    d. protection from radiation exposure

13. A PACS is useful for what within a hospital?
    a. making images available to multiple computers
    b. monitoring of radiation exposure
    c. positioning of sedated animals
    d. intensifying the screen image

14. What items are included in full radiation protection?
    a. lined fingerless gloves, thyroid shield, gown
    b. chaps, gown, thyroid shield
    c. cap, gown, gloves
    d. full gloves, gown, thyroid shield

15. Which tissues are most sensitive to radiation damage?
    a. gastrointestinal tract
    b. reproducing cells
    c. renal
    d. brain

16. What stage of pregnancy poses the greatest risk for radiation exposure?
    a. 0–6 weeks
    b. 10–15 weeks
    c. 20–30 weeks
    d. the last trimester

17. How often should protective lead-lined equipment be checked for damage?
    a. weekly
    b. monthly
    c. every 6 months
    d. every 12 months

18. In what procedures would a flexible endoscope be used?
    a. arthroscopy
    b. rhinoscopy
    c. female cystoscopy
    d. bronchoscopy

19. When performing an MRI, what items should not be in the room?
    a. any ferromagnetic object
    b. all anesthetics
    c. urinary catheters
    d. intravenous catheters

20. What imaging modality can be used when the metabolic process needs to be evaluated?
    a. fluoroscopy
    b. endoscopy
    c. ultrasound
    d. scintigraphy

21. Which imaging technique uses contrast media to visualize the spinal cord?
    a. ultrasound
    b. myelography
    c. CT
    d. DICOM

22. Which imaging modality uses magnets to produce images inside the body?
    a. ultrasound
    b. CT
    c. MRI
    d. CCD

23. How do x-rays differ from visible light?
    a. their longer wavelengths
    b. the amount of heat produced
    c. their faster moving electrons
    d. their lower energy

24. Where is a Bucky grid found?
    a. In a cabinet beneath the x-ray table
    b. Outside the diagnostic room
    c. Inside the chest, just below the sternum
    d. At the epiphyseal plate in growing animals

25. What is gadolinium most commonly used for?
    a. decrease scatter radiation
    b. skin contact during ultrasound
    c. contrast media in MRI
    d. preventing urination during CT

26. Which part of an ultrasound machine emits a series of sound pulses and receives the returning echoes?
    a. the computer
    b. the transducer
    c. transduction gel
    d. the time gain compensator

27. What type of patient preparation is required to achieve a diagnostic ultrasound?
    a. heavy sedation
    b. enema and 24-hour fasting
    c. shaving the hair coat
    d. application of a waterless shampoo

28. What would be an example of a negative contrast agent?
    a. air
    b. barium
    c. transducer gel
    d. meglumine

29. The distance from the target to the recording surface with radiographs is called what?
    a. focal film distance
    b. penumbra distance
    c. radiographic source distance
    d. source-image distance

30. Which type of digital radiograph uses a scanner laser beam to produce an image?
    a. MRI
    b. CR
    c. CCD
    d. DR

31. What type of electrons are produced by the cathode?
    a. negative

b. positive
    c. neutral
    d. black

32. What is the unit of measurement for the sound frequency produced by the transducer in ultrasounds?
    a. Sieverts
    b. Rems
    c. Megahertz
    d. Gray

33. Which imaging modality uses an x-ray tube that freely rotates around a patient, creating a dataset of images?
    a. fluoroscopy
    b. CT
    c. MRI
    d. CCD

34. When doing a contrast study of the GI tract to identify a perforation, what contrast agent should be avoided?
    a. air
    b. meglumine
    c. barium
    d. diatrizoate

35. Which imaging technique can produce a continual stream of images making cardiac and motility studies easier?
    a. endoscopy
    b. CT
    c. MRI
    d. fluoroscopy

36. What is the typical focal film distance with dental radiographs?
    a. 6 inches
    b. 12 inches
    c. 22 inches
    d. 40 inches

37. Which teeth's images are produced using the parallel technique when taking dental images?
    a. mandibular premolars
    b. maxillary incisors
    c. all molars
    d. maxillary canines

38. Under what conditions the bisecting angle technique is used?
    a. the teeth are immature
    b. there is excessive crowding of the mandibular teeth
    c. there is a significant gingival recession
    d. when the film cannot be placed parallel to the tooth

39. Which position is preferred for radiographs of the maxillary incisors?
    a. dorsal
    b. ventral
    c. sternal
    d. lateral

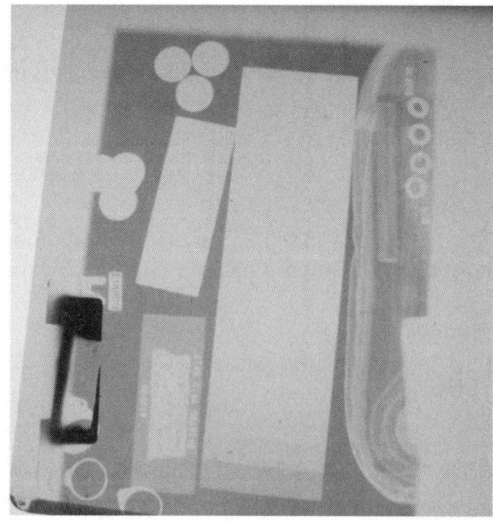

1. Why does the radiograph show a low density?

_____

_____

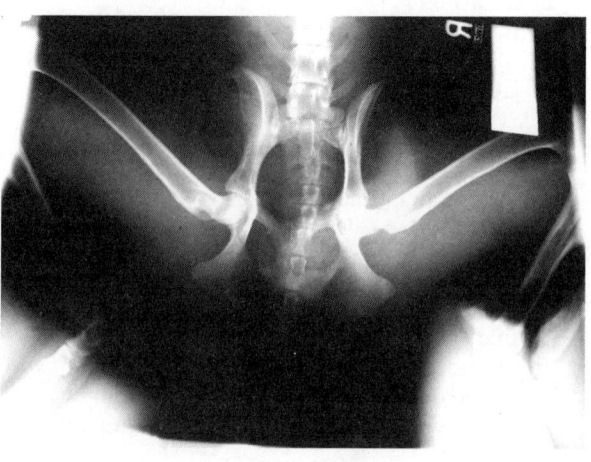

3. What are the white areas at the corners of the radiograph, and why is this a problem?

_____

_____

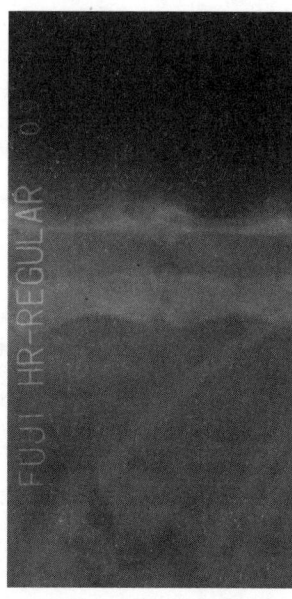

2. Is this a low- or high-contrast film?

_____

_____

4. The whitest area is the thickest or thinnest portion of the step wedge.

_____

_____

5. From left to right, what tissue densities are represented in each area?

_____

_____

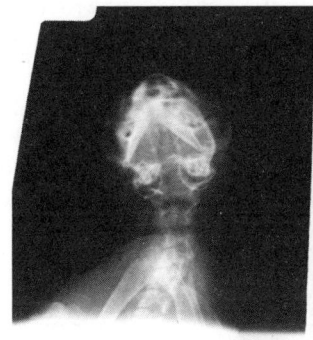 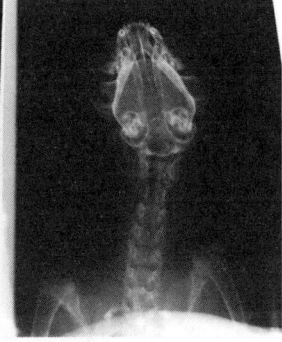

6. Which skull has the highest contrast?

_____

_____

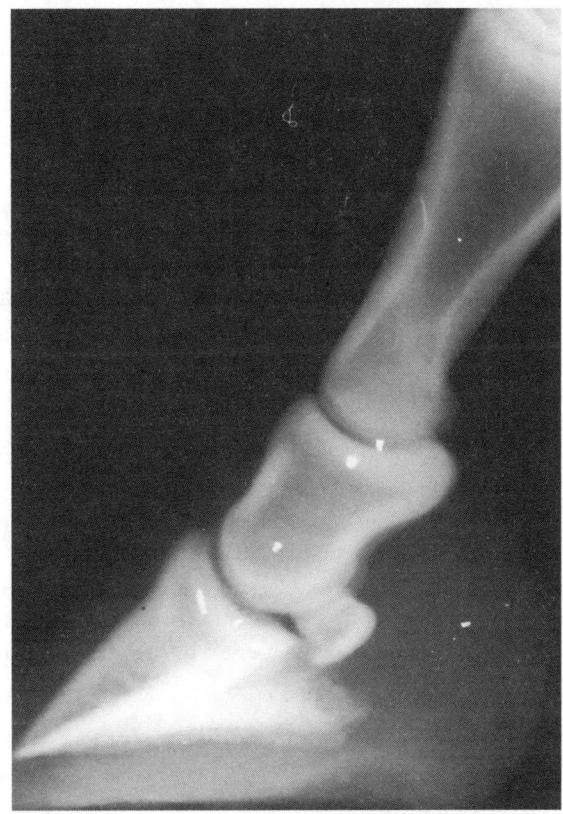

7. The small white circles on this hoof are caused by what density of an object?

_____

_____

12 Avian and Exotic Animal Care and Nursing

LEARNING OBJECTIVES

After reviewing this chapter, the reader will be able to:

- State the general characteristics of mice, rats, hamsters, gerbils, guinea pigs, chinchillas, rabbits, and ferrets.
- Discuss husbandry and principles of sanitation for small mammals.
- Describe techniques for general nursing care of rodents, rabbits, and ferrets.
- Describe techniques used for diagnosing and treating disease in small mammals.
- Describe the unique features of the anatomy of birds and the basic biology of common reptile species.
- Discuss the basic behavior of birds, reptiles, and amphibians.
- Discuss the basics of client education, husbandry, and nutrition for the avian, reptilian, and amphibian species.
- Describe how to obtain a complete and thorough history of avian, reptilian, and amphibian patients.
- Explain the different capture and restraint techniques used for birds, reptiles, and amphibians.
- Identify methods of sample collection for laboratory analysis.
- Describe how to obtain high-quality diagnostic images of avian, reptilian, and amphibian patients.
- Discuss nursing care and supportive therapy techniques for avian, reptilian, and amphibian patients.
- Identify and discuss some of the common diseases of avian, reptilian, and amphibian patients of a veterinary clinic.

LABELING—AVIAN RESPIRATORY SYSTEM

Identify the elements in this diagram of the avian respiratory system, lateral view.

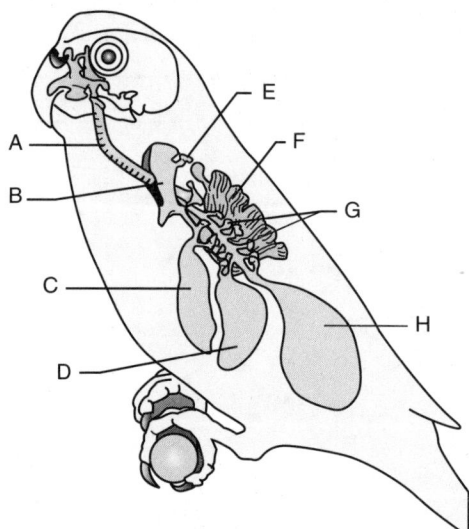

A. _____	E. _____
B. _____	F. _____
C. _____	G. _____
D. _____	H. _____

LABELING—FEATHERS

Identify the types of feathers shown.

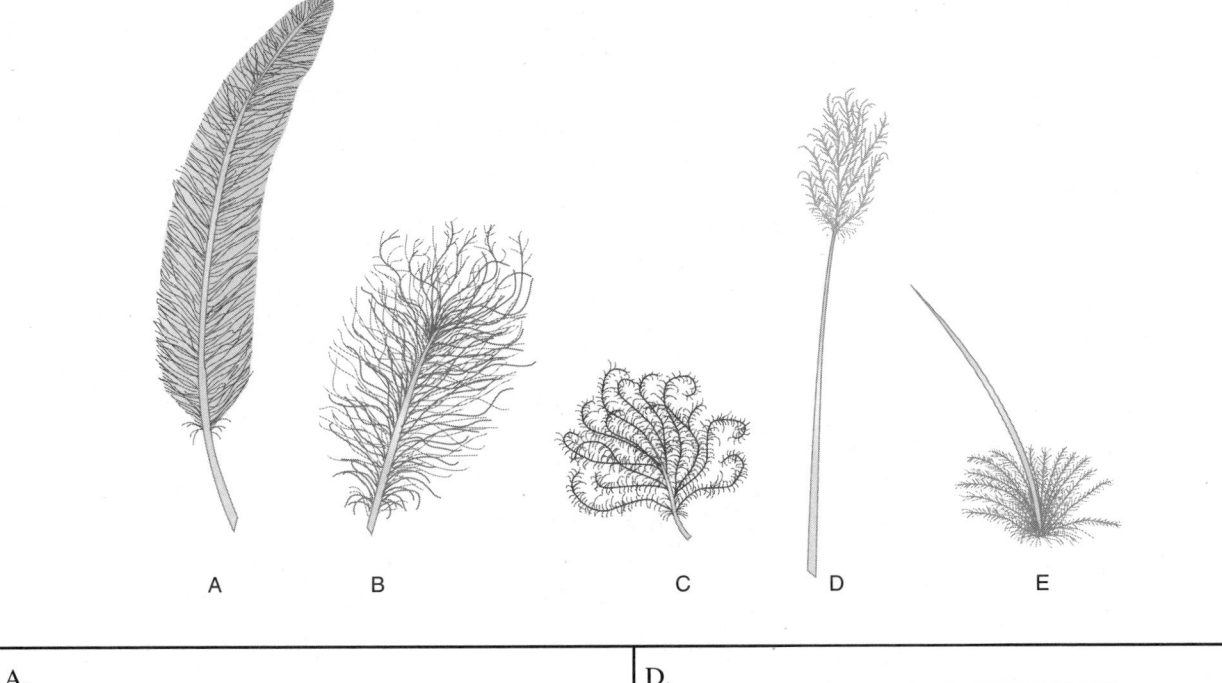

A   B   C   D   E

A. _____	D. _____
B. _____	E. _____
C. _____	

SHORT ANSWER, FILL IN THE BLANK, AND LISTS

1. Signs of respiratory distress in a bird include the following:

   A. _____

   B. _____

   C. _____

   D. _____

   E. _____

   F. _____

   G. _____

2. Regarding sites for the administration of fluid and medication in lizards:

   A. When handling reptiles, wear latex or examination gloves to protect yourself from exposure to _____.

   B. The most common routes are usually _____ sites.

   C. A _____ feeding tube is generally used when force-feeding most reptile and amphibian species.

   D. A _____ feeding tube is generally used when force-feeding most avian species.

   E. Chelonians, lizards, and snakes commonly present in emergencies as a result of _____ injuries.

3. List the common venipuncture sites for the following species:

   Chelonians _____

   Lizards _____

   Snakes _____

MATCHING

Match the disease or conditions with the description.

1. _____ *Bordetella bronchiseptica*	A. Gum infection common in ferrets
2. _____ Canine distemper	B. Zoonotic disease that causes psittacosis in humans and avian chlamydiosis in avian species
3. _____ Coccidia	C. Cutaneous bacterial infection
4. _____ Heatstroke	D. Rabbit ear mite
5. _____ Dysecdysis	E. Common endoparasite in rabbits
6. _____ Pododermatitis	F. Difficulty in shedding the skin in reptiles
7. _____ *Mesocricetus auratus*	G. Pressure necrosis of the plantar surface of the metatarsal area seen in obese rabbits
8. _____ West Nile virus	H. Herpetic virus seen in psittacids
9. _____ Chlamydiosis	I. Sensitivity to light
10. _____ *Psoroptes*	J. Susceptibility in guinea pigs
11. _____ Phototoxicity	K. Chinchillas prone to this with increased humidity
12. _____ Pacheco disease	L. Mosquito-borne disease that primarily infects horses, humans, and birds
13. _____ Red leg	M. Golden hamster
14. _____ Periodontal disease	N. Fatal disease of ferrets

MULTIPLE CHOICE

1. Which of the following is true concerning the respiratory system of birds?
   a. Air enters the respiratory system through the nares and continues over an operculum.
   b. An epiglottis is present.
   c. Lobes and alveoli are present so the lungs can inflate.
   d. The diaphragm assists in the inspiration of air through the extension of the intracostal joints.

2. Which of the following is true concerning airflow in birds?
   a. Mouth breathing is normal.
   b. The unpaired air sac is the interclavicular air sac.
   c. The respiratory tract cannot communicate with the long bones.
   d. Gas exchange occurs in the air sacs.

3. Concerning the special senses of birds, which statement is not true?
   a. Birds have the traditional five senses: seeing, hearing, feeling, smelling, and tasting.
   b. Hearing is done through the coordination of the five bones of the inner ear.
   c. Bird vision is very acute, and birds can perceive color.
   d. Birds have more taste buds than mammals.

4. Which common bird toxin can result in vomiting, diarrhea, blood in the stools, and increased respiration?
   a. hydrocarbon-based compounds
   b. tobacco
   c. matches
   d. household cleaners

5. Which statement regarding reptilian biology is true?
   a. Like birds, reptiles have a diaphragm to separate the thoracic and abdominal cavities.
   b. There is one visceral cavity, called the coelom.
   c. Reptiles can generate their own body heat.
   d. Reptile excrement contains two components—urates and feces.

6. Which of the following is true concerning examining or restraining amphibians?
   a. Wearing unpowdered gloves can help avoid dehydration in the patient
   b. Their skin is very thick and does not easily absorb substance through it
   c. They can be scruffed for restraint
   d. They should never be anesthetized

7. Which of the following is true concerning husbandry of reptiles?
   a. The only purpose of cage furniture is to provide a hiding place.
   b. Hot rocks and sizzle stones can cause thermal burns.
   c. Supplemental UV lighting is only needed if they are not housed near a window.
   d. Wood chips are an excellent bedding surface.

8. Which of the following is true concerning amphibian care and feeding?
   a. Temperature, pH, salinity, and hardness of water should be checked regularly.
   b. Nitrogenous waste buildup and disinfectant residues are easily tolerated.
   c. Water filtration is not required.
   d. They can easily break down excess disinfectants left in a cage.

9. Feather mutilation and plucking are common behaviors of which bird species?
   a. cockatoos
   b. pigeons
   c. canaries
   d. budgies

10. The fecal slide you are examining shows gram-positive bacterial flora and some yeast. You are likely examining the feces of which bird grouping?
    a. Captive raptors
    b. Domesticated Galliformes
    c. Grain- and fruit-eating Psittaciformes
    d. Fresh-water Anseriformes

11. Where is the diastema found in rats?
    a. under the skin
    b. between the toes on the back feet
    c. between the oral cavity and the incisors
    d. in the inguinal space of males

12. The Harderian gland is located near which sensory organ in rats?
    ___ a. the mouth
    ___ b. the eye
    ___ c. the ears
    ___ d. the skin

13. Which animals are found under the classification of lagomorph?
    ___ a. rabbits
    ___ b. mice
    ___ c. parrots
    ___ d. terrestrial amphibians

14. The haustra in rabbits is found in what part of their digestive tract?
    ___ a. stomach
    ___ b. duodenum
    ___ c. cecum
    ___ d. colon

15. What is the average core body temperature of an adult bird?
    a. 25°C–30°C (77°F–86°F)
    b. 32°C–36°C (90°F–99°F)
    c. 38°C–42°C (105°F–109°F)
    d. 45°C–50°C (113°F–122°F)

16. What is a blood feather?
    a. new, growing feathers that are not full sized
    b. established feathers from this year's molt
    c. normal plumage
    d. dropped feathers at the time of molting

17. What is the purpose of the uropygial gland?
    a. to aid in the digestion of grains
    b. to produce tears
    c. lubricate the oviduct for easier egg passage
    d. to waterproof feathers during preening

18. Where on the wing are the flight feathers located in birds?
    a. over the body near the base of the wing
    b. the tail
    c. outer edge of the wing
    d. ringed around the neck

19. In birds, which digestive organ is comparable to the stomach of mammals?
    a. haustra
    b. proventriculus
    c. ventriculus
    d. cloaca

20. Which muscle group in birds supports flight?
    a. quadriceps
    b. proctodeum
    c. pectorals
    d. mandibular

21. In most birds, ovulation to egg laying takes approximately how much time?
    a. 15 hours
    b. 30 hours
    c. 45 hours
    d. 60 hours

22. How are avian RBCs different from mammals?
    a. They have a green pigment rather than a red pigment.
    b. They are produced in the lymph nodes, not the bone marrow.
    c. They are oval and nucleated.
    d. They are phagocytic.

23. What restraint device is preferred when capturing pet birds?
    a. Bare hands are fine.
    b. Wildlife gloves.
    c. A net.
    d. A big fluffy towel.

24. Dysecdysis describes which problem in captive reptiles?
    a. shedding
    b. bone metabolism
    c. defecation
    d. egg passage

25. What tool can be used to rim an overlong beak in birds?
    a. regular toenail trimmers
    b. handheld nail file
    c. sanding stone
    d. handheld rotary grinder

26. What is the best means of permanent identification for birds?
    a. leg bands
    b. microchips
    c. painting the toenails
    d. a collar

27. What handling challenge is presented by box turtles?
    a. They are always covered in algae making them slippery.
    b. They have long necks and can reach around to bite you easily.
    c. They have a hinged plastron and can tuck themselves into their shells.
    d. The plastron is very fragile and can break with ordinary handling.

28. What type of diet is preferred for snakes?
    a. herbivorous, primarily grains
    b. fructivorous
    c. omnivore
    d. carnivore, whole prey

29. What type of diet is preferred by most aquatic turtles?
    a. herbivorous, primarily grains
    b. fructivorous
    c. omnivore
    d. carnivore, whole prey

30. What are the primary causes of diseases in exotic or atypical animals?
    a. poor husbandry and improper diet
    b. domestication that occurs too quickly
    c. lack of a social group
    d. insufficient opportunities for breeding

31. What problem can be seen in gerbils who are housed in conditions where the temperature can fall below 8°C (46°F)?
    a. aggression
    b. permissive hibernation
    c. increased appetite 2–3× above normal
    d. hyperthermia to compensate

32. Which rodent species has a dietary requirement for vitamin C?
    a. mice
    b. hamsters
    c. guinea pigs
    d. rabbits

33. A gerbil has a midventral dark-orange sebaceous gland. What is its primary purpose?
    a. preening
    b. territorial marking
    c. sexual differentiation
    d. prevention of anal gland impaction

34. What is the average lifespan for a ferret?
    a. 2–3 years
    b. 3–4 years
    c. 5–8 years
    d. 9–10 years

35. When sexing ferrets, a male can be identified by this placement of their preputial opening.
    a. below the anal opening
    b. above the anal opening
    c. on the ventral abdomen
    d. on the dorsal abdomen

36. What causes estrogen toxicity in female ferrets?
    a. persistent estrus cycles
    b. adrenal tumors
    c. distemper infection
    d. being spayed too early

37. When administering oral antibiotics to certain rodents, what can happen if the normal gram-positive flora are destroyed?
    a. fecal impaction
    b. psittacosis
    c. enterotoxemia
    d. periodontal disease

38. What is the top shell of a chelonian called?
    a. squamata
    b. carapace
    c. plastron
    d. testudines

39. A diurnal animal is active during what parts of the day?
    a. early morning and early evening
    b. late morning once it has warmed up
    c. during the daytime
    d. during the evening

40. Which mammal species is known to be coprophagic?
    a. rats and mice
    b. hamsters
    c. ferrets
    d. rabbits

41. Birds that are anisodactyl have how many toes, pointed in what orientation?
    a. 3 toes pointed forward, and 1 pointed back
    b. 2 toes pointed forward, and 2 pointed back

    c. 1 toe pointed forward, and 2 pointed back
    d. 1 toe pointed forward, and 3 pointed back

42. Flying birds have what kind of bones that make them lighter?
    a. continually growing
    b. pneumatic
    c. compact
    d. osteomalacia

43. Terrestrial tortoises eat what type of diet?
    a. herbivore
    b. carnivore
    c. fructivore
    d. omnivore

44. What is the typical treatment if a bird has ingested lead or zinc from their toys or cages?
    a. induction of vomiting
    b. chelation therapy
    c. administration of activated charcoal
    d. unfortunately, there is no treatment

PHOTO QUIZ

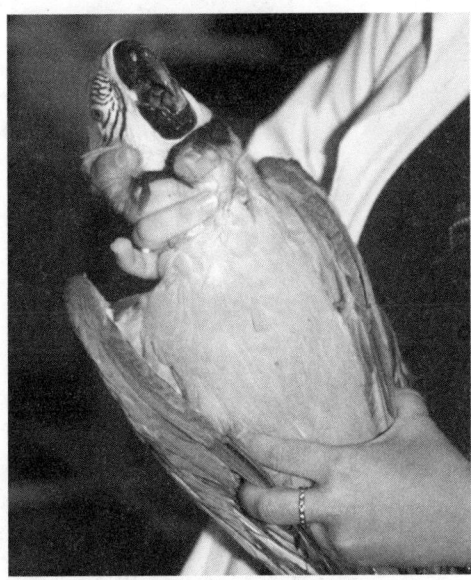

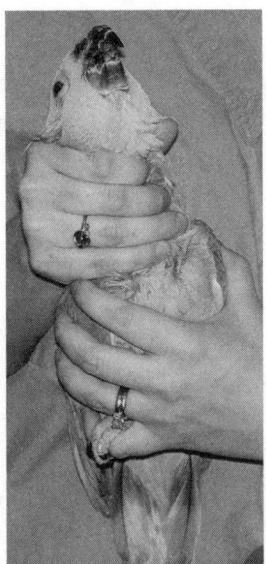

1. Is the restraint of this bird correct? Why or why not?

   _____

   _____

2. Is this the correct restraint for this parrot? Why or why not?

   _____

   _____

79

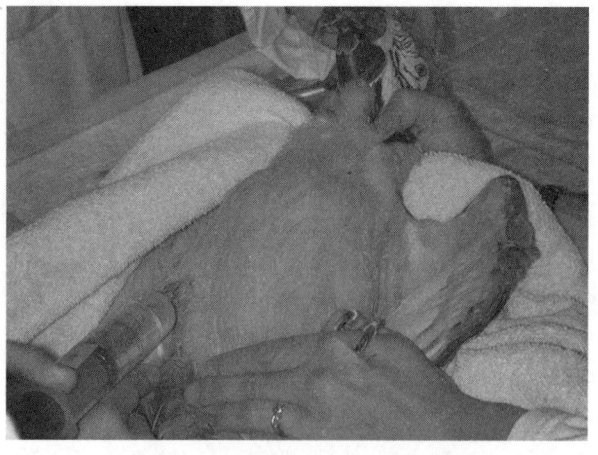

3. The site for these subcutaneous fluids is _____

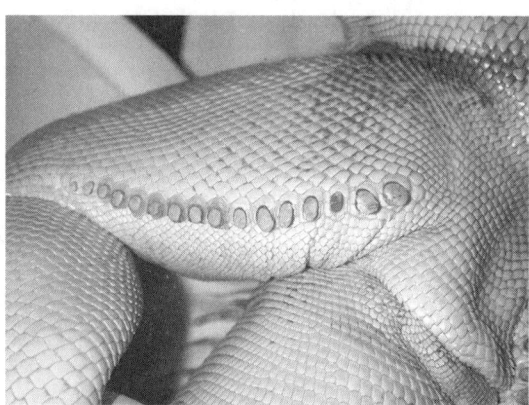

4. What are these structures called in lizards?

_____

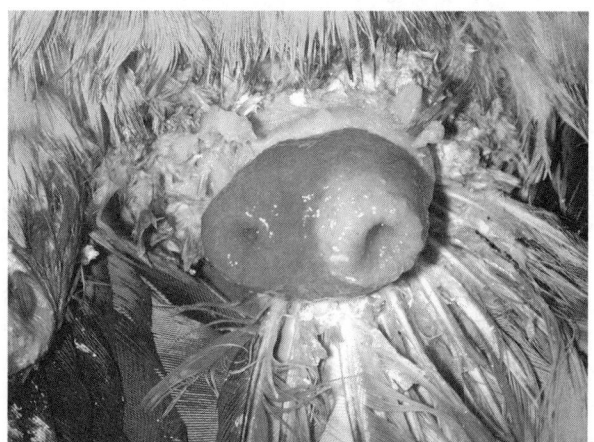

5. This image demonstrates what condition in birds?

_____ .

6. This snake's skin and eyes are turning an opaque blue color. What is about to happen?

_____

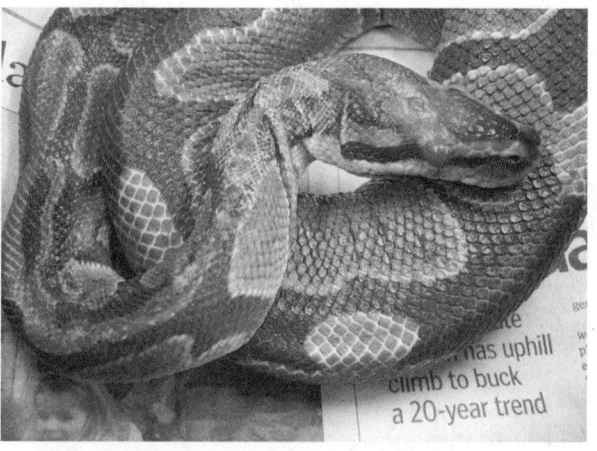

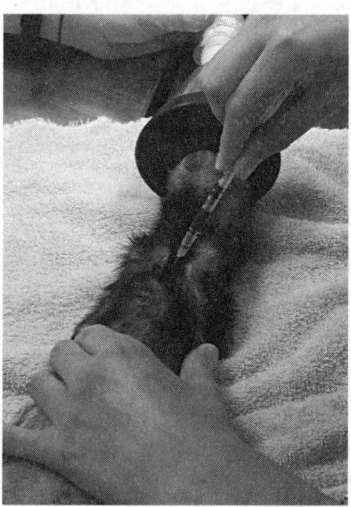

7. Name the blood vessel being used for the blood collection on this ferret.

_____

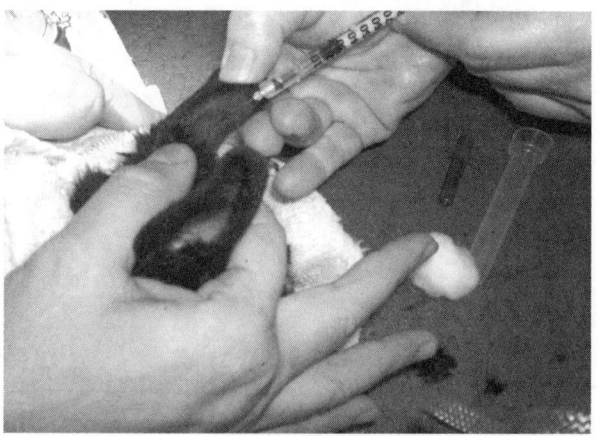

8. Name the blood vessel being used for the blood collection on this rabbit.

_____

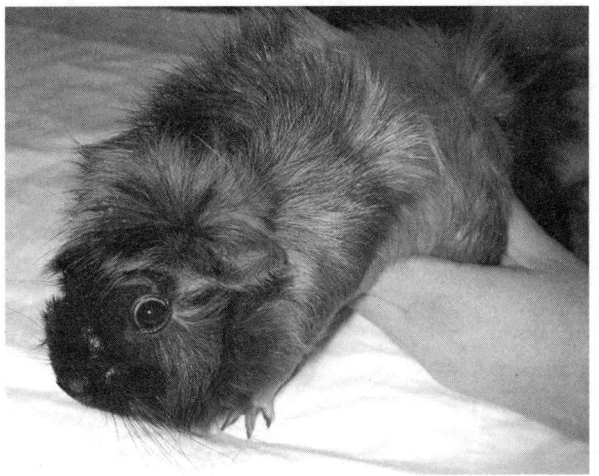

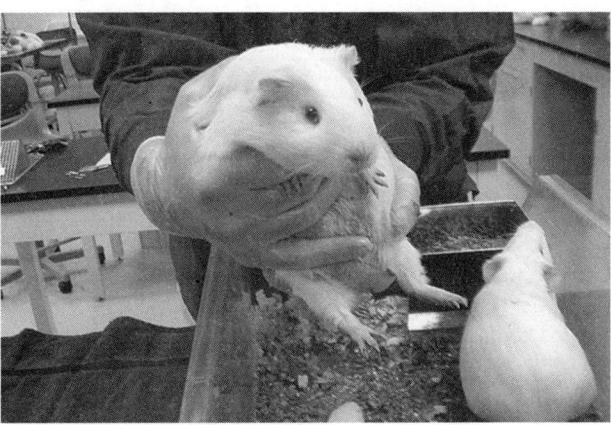

9. Name this breed of guinea pig.

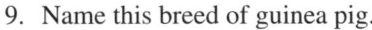

10. Is this the correct method for the removal of this guinea pig from a cage? Why or why not?

_____

_____

CASE SCENARIO

Please complete the following table with the requested information.

Mammal	Classification	Lifespan
Rabbit		
Ferret		
Mouse		
Rat		
Hamster		
Gerbil		
Guinea pig		
Chinchilla		

Please complete the following table with the requested information.

Birds			
Feather types	Contour	Coverts	Down
Type of bones		X	X
Choana location		X	X
Number of air sacs		X	X
Proventriculus		X	X
Ventriculus		X	X
Cloaca location		X	X
Female reproductive tract		X	X
Columella location		X	X
Reasons for biting			
Behavior problems			X
Microchip location		X	X
Zoonotic diseases			

Please complete the following table with the requested information.

Reptiles	Order	Most Common Pets	Shedding Pattern	Diet Requirements
Snakes				
Lizards				
Turtles				
Tortoises				

Please complete the following table with the requested information.

Amphibian	Order	Venipuncture Sites
Frogs		
Toads		
Salamanders		
Newts		X
Sirens		X
Caecilians		X

13 | Large Animal Nursing and Husbandry

LEARNING OBJECTIVES

After reviewing this chapter, the reader will be able to:
- Describe the general husbandry needs of large animals.
- Describe restraint methods used with large animals.
- Explain and demonstrate routine procedures used in grooming and foot care.
- Discuss the techniques used in general nursing care of large animals.
- Compare and contrast various routes of administration of medication in large animals.
- Identify and describe various methods of sample collection for laboratory analysis.

FILL IN THE BLANK

1. A _____ is any dietary component that provides some essential nutrient or serves some other function.

2. _____ are feeds made up of most or all of the plant.

3. _____ is the most common grain fed to livestock.

4. Because calves are born essentially _____, provision of colostrum shortly after birth is critically important.

5. For calves with fluid loss because of neonatal enteritis, _____ solutions are commonly offered as a means to provide additional fluid therapy.

6. Silage is not commonly fed to horses because of their sensitivity to the _____ and _____ potentially found in silage.

7. _____ produces less dust and may be better for horses recovering from respiratory allergies or pneumonia.

8. Pig diets consist primarily of _____, along with energy, protein, mineral, and vitamin supplements.

9. Goats may be used for _____, _____, or _____ production.

10. Physical assessment of production animals may include observations of hair coat, _____, hydration status, manure consistency, and attitude.

11. Black walnut shavings can cause _____ when the horse stands in the shavings.

12. Topical fly sprays that contain _____, _____, or _____ are safest for sick horses.

13. The horse's hoof is cleaned with a hoof pick by removing debris from the lateral and central sulci, starting at the ____ and working toward the _____, and then from the rest of the hoof.

14. Common methods of identification of individual poultry include _____, ____wing ____, and _____.

15. An alert horse has its ears _____.

MATCHING

Select the proper male or female name for the following animals.

1. _____ Adult intact male ovine	A. Gilt
2. _____ Male adult bovine	B. Bull
3. _____ Adult female porcine	C. Piglet
4. _____ Young female porcine before farrowing	D. Doe
5. _____ Adult female ovine	E. Lamb
6. _____ Adult intact male caprine	F. Sow
7. _____ Castrated male porcine	G. Heifer
8. _____ Female adult bovine	H. Buck/Ram
9. _____ Castrated male ovines/caprines	I. Boar
10. _____ Adult female caprine	J. Cow
11. _____ Male castrated bovine	K. Wether
12. _____ Young ovine	L. Billy/Ram
13. _____ Female young adult bovine	M. Steer
14. _____ Young porcine	N. Ewe
15. _____ Intact adult male porcine	O. Barrow

MULTIPLE CHOICE

1. What type of fly repellents should not be applied to debilitated horses?
   a. Permethrins
   b. Pyrethrins
   c. Organophosphates
   d. Citronella

2. Using the standard 9-point body condition score, what number is used to represent an emaciated animal?
   a. 1
   b. 3
   c. 6
   d. 9

3. What type of diet do pigs typically eat?
   a. Carnivore
   b. Herbivore
   c. Insectivore
   d. Omnivore

4. What grooming tool can be used to remove dried sweat and mud from a horse's face?
   a. Pick
   b. Metal curry comb
   c. Rubber curry comb
   d. Metal comb

5. When would thrush be expected to occur in horse feet?
   a. Hot, dry conditions
   b. Infrequent cleaning
   c. After viral laminitis
   d. When fed too much silage

6. Any angry or fearful horse will often do what with their ears?
   a. Swivel them around to monitor the situation
   b. Prick them forward
   c. Pin them back
   d. Have them pointed in different directions

7. When approaching a horse, from what side and direction is recommended?
   a. From the front and slightly on the left side
   b. From straight ahead in the middle
   c. From directly behind them and on the right side
   d. From either side at the shoulder

8. When restraining a horse for the veterinarian, what side should you be standing on?
   a. Opposite side
   b. Same side
   c. Directly in front of them
   d. Directly behind them

9. What tool is used to measure the specific gravity of the colostrum?
   a. Refractometer
   b. Hydrometer
   c. Colostrometer
   d. Hygrometer

10. What term describes the minimum length of time from the administration of the last dose of a medication until the animal is slaughtered?
   a. Gestation
   b. Incubation
   c. Chemical
   d. Withdrawal

11. Which species has a gestation of 283 days?
   a. Horse
   b. Cattle
   c. Goat
   d. Pig

12. Which species has the shortest gestation at 114 days (3 months, 3 weeks, 3 days)
   a. Horse
   b. Cattle
   c. Goat
   d. Pig

13. At what age are meat chickens typically sent to slaughter?
   a. 16–24 weeks
   b. 6–8 months
   c. 10–12 months
   d. After their first molt

14. What restraint device can be used on dairy cows who tend to kick milkers?
   a. Tail jack
   b. Hobbles
   c. Ear twitch
   d. Nose ring

15. Which restraint device is used almost exclusively on beef cattle?
   a. Hobbles
   b. Tail jack
   c. Squeeze chute
   d. Nose ring

16. Forages are composed of what part(s) of the plants?
   a. Flowering tops
   b. Stalks and stems
   c. Roots and stems
   d. All of the plant

17. What type of plants can be used as forages?
   a. Grasses and legumes
   b. Hardwood saplings and shoots
   c. Compost and silage
   d. Anything green and growing

18. What type of digestive tract do cattle, sheep, and goats have?
   a. Monogastric
   b. Enlarged cecum
   c. Ruminant
   d. Hindgut fermentation

19. Pregastric fermentation occurs in which chamber of a ruminant?
   a. Rumen
   b. Reticulum
   c. Omasum
   d. Abomasum

20. Which form of forage is the least digestible?
   a. Hay
   b. Straw
   c. Silage
   d. Concentrates

21. Silage is stored using what type of fermentation?
   a. Pickling
   b. Drying
   c. Oxygenation
   d. Green chop

22. Cereal grains are fed as concentrates due to their large amounts of what nutrient?
   a. Lignin
   b. Fats
   c. Proteins
   d. Starch

23. What is the most common oilseed crop fed to livestock?
   a. Canola meal
   b. Cottonseed meal
   c. Soybean meal
   d. Peanut seed meal

24. How are dairy cattle house?
   a. Breed
   b. Production stage
   c. Sex
   d. Preferred feed type

25. What type of beef cattle operations focuses on calf production?
    a. Cow-calf
    b. Cattle feeding
    c. Dairy production
    d. Feedlots

26. What type of problems can be indicated by lack of a suckle reflex in newborn calves?
    a. Antigammaglobulinemia
    b. Acidosis from dystocia
    c. Insufficient colostrum production by the cow
    d. Respiratory alkalinity

27. What is scours in young cattle?
    a. A hacking cough
    b. Hyperthermia
    c. Enteritis
    d. Biting at the bars of the cages causing breathing difficulties

28. What nutrient does beet pulp provide to horses in their diets?
    a. Protein
    b. Fat
    c. Water-soluble vitamins
    d. Fermentable fiber

29. What type of digestive tract do horses have?
    a. Monogastric
    b. Hindgut fermenters
    c. Ruminants
    d. Multigastric

30. With pigs, how are animals in the farrowing operation housed?
    a. Group housed by age
    b. Group housed by sex
    c. Individually house
    d. Open housed

31. What type of feed is most often used with pigs?
    a. High fiber, low protein
    b. Concentrates with supplements
    c. Moderate fiber with supplements
    d. Pelleted hay with a vitamin premix

32. What type of diet is typically fed to sheep?
    a. Forage plus vitamin-mineral supplements
    b. Pelleted concentrates
    c. Silage
    d. Complete and balanced kibble

33. What effect does lactation have on the energy requirements for goats?
    a. None, they require the same as meat goats
    b. Slight increase that can be met with increased forage
    c. Slight increase that can be met with added vitamin-mineral supplementation
    d. Substantial increase that requires energy supplementation

34. What method is used to subjectively quantify subcutaneous body fat reserves?
    a. Tape measure at the widest part of the chest
    b. Weight
    c. Body condition score
    d. Frame size

35. What bedding has been associated with laminitis in horses?
    a. Black walnut shavings
    b. Pine shavings
    c. Fresh leaves
    d. Sand

36. What method of exercise is best for foals?
    a. A treadmill
    b. Running freely alongside the mare
    c. Lunging using a halter
    d. Retractable leash alongside the side of the road

37. What PPE should be worn when applying treatments for thrush to a horse's hoof?
    a. Heavy petroleum jelly application
    b. A 2% iodine solution prewash
    c. Latex or nitrile examination gloves
    d. Full face mask and surgical gloves

38. Which of these breeds is heavily muscled and used for beef production?
    a. Holstein
    b. Angus
    c. Jersey
    d. Suffolk

39. Which of these breeds is efficient at milk production and used in dairy production?
    a. Texas longhorn
    b. Brahman
    c. Guernsey
    d. Herford

40. What type of breeding programs are used with beef breeds?
    a. Allowing bulls in the fields within heat females
    b. Exclusively artificial insemination
    c. Individually housing females with easy access to a bull
    d. Field confinement until they are receptive then individually housed

41. When does an ewe need to be bred to get spring lambs?
    a. The previous spring
    b. The previous summer
    c. The previous fall
    d. The previous winter

42. What is the purpose of an elastrator?
    a. Dehorning
    b. Castration
    c. Increasing growth rates
    d. Decreasing the requirement for concentrates in the diet

43. Mohair fiber is obtained from which livestock animal?
    a. Sheep
    b. Cattle
    c. Horses
    d. Goats

44. At what age are pigs typically sent to market?
    a. 12 weeks
    b. 5–6 months
    c. 8–10 months
    d. After 12 months of age

45. What environmental condition is a problem with newborn piglets?
    a. Hypothermia
    b. Low humidity
    c. Hypoglycemia
    d. Crowding

46. Poultry refers to what type of livestock animals?
    a. Dairy and beef cattle
    b. Meat and wool sheep
    c. Ducks and geese
    d. Meat and fat pigs

47. At what point are laying hens typically sent to slaughter?
    a. 20–24 weeks
    b. After 12 months of age
    c. After their first molt
    d. After their second molt

48. What happens to laying hens in the winter when the days become shorter than 14 hours?
    a. They go into pseudohibernation
    b. Egg production falls
    c. They become broody
    d. They become hyperthermic

49. In dual-purpose poultry, what are those two purposes?
    a. Feather production and manure
    b. Eggs and feathers
    c. Meat and eggs
    d. Wool and meat

50. What site is used for an IM injection in a horse?
    a. Lateral aspect of the neck
    b. Along the thoracic spine
    c. In the rear leg
    d. Ventral abdomen

CASE SCENARIO

You are going to a smaller livestock farm in your area for routine yearly examinations of the animals. They have dairy cattle (two different breeds, both cows), dairy goats (one breed, three goats), one pot-bellied pig, one donkey, one miniature horse, and two sheep raised for their hair.

For each of these species, provide the purpose that they are typically raised for, what type of digestive tract they have, common housing considerations, common restraint methods, and sites for injections.

Species	Purpose	Digestion	Housing	Common Restraint Methods	Injection Sites
Dairy cattle					
Dairy goats					
Pot-bellied pig	ornamental!				
Donkey					
Miniature horse	ornamental!				
Sheep					

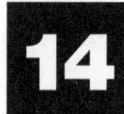 **Hospice, Grief, and Pet Loss**

LEARNING OBJECTIVES

After reviewing this chapter, the reader will be able to:

- Describe the human-animal bond.
- Identify the differences between palliative care, respite care, and hospice care.
- Explain the role of euthanasia in veterinary medicine.
- Describe the stages of grief.
- Describe the effects of patient loss on the veterinary team.
- Explain the effects of compounded loss on owners and the veterinary team.
- Demonstrate knowledge of grief counseling.
- Identify and discuss differing ways of memorializing pets.

FILL IN THE BLANK

1. Palliative care is directed at _____ of life, not necessarily the quantity of life.

2. The most effective pain control utilizes a _____ approach.

3. To help identify patients who are masking their pain, _____ _____ _____ can be used.

4. What would be examples of set points in determining quality of life?

   a. _____

   b. _____

   c. _____

   d. _____

   e. _____

5. What three mechanisms are involved in a patient's death?

   a. _____

   b. _____

   c. _____

6. What physical signs can be used to confirm death?

   a. _____

   b. _____

   c. _____

   d. _____

   e. _____

   f. _____

7. What are some ways of expressing condolences for a loss to a client?

   a. _____

   b. _____

   c. _____

   d. _____

8. What types of memorials are available after the loss of a pet?

   a. _____

   b. _____

   c. _____

   d. _____

   e. _____

   f. _____

   g. _____

9. What are some ways in which owners can have relationships with their pets?

   a. _____

   b. _____

   c. _____

   d. _____

10. What type of support materials are helpful to grieving clients?

   a. _____

   b. _____

   c. _____

   d. _____

   e. _____

   f. _____

MATCHING

Dr. Elisabeth Kübler-Ross described the stages of grief. Match the stage to the signs typically seen.

Stage	Signs
1. _____ Denial	A. Able to recall good times with a smile rather than sorrow
2. _____ Bargaining	B. Clients who never have another pet do not reach this stage
3. _____ Anger	C. Deep sadness
4. _____ Guilt	D. Feeling an empty space even with family and friends near
5. _____ Sorrow	E. Blaming the veterinary teams for their inability to save a pet
6. _____ Resolution	F. Attempting to buy more time with the pet
7. _____ Loneliness	G. A coping mechanism that serves to cushion the mind
8. _____ Replacement	H. Unproductive and debilitating emotion

MULTIPLE CHOICE

1. In the past century, where has the focus of veterinary medicine evolved from?
   a. Diagnosing to treating
   b. Food animals to companion animals
   c. Mammals to reptiles and birds
   d. Cruelty prevention to TNR

2. When treating all patients, the primary responsibility of the veterinary team is to whom?
   a. The owner
   b. The bonded person
   c. The practice
   d. The patient

3. What do we know regarding the human-animal bond?
   a. The bond is the same for everyone in the family
   b. The bond can vary between different people in the house
   c. The bond exists only between companion animals
   d. The bond can prevent adequate care

4. When building a bond with a patient in the hospital, it is important to remember what?
   a. Pets always behave the same in all situations
   b. Breed behaviors are consistent
   c. Pets can act differently with different people
   d. Chemical sedation is not required for routine or advanced care

5. What is the primary reason animals are left at animal shelters?
   a. Expensive medical problems
   b. They are old and the family wants a new pet
   c. The breed is no longer en vogue
   d. Behavioral problems

6. What additional concerns do we need to be able to address when working with service dogs or assistance animals?
   a. Treatment that may temporarily incapacitate the animal
   b. Pain medication is not able to be used
   c. The cost of advanced treatment options
   d. The necessity of separating the animal and the owner for treatment for their safety

7. What actions by the hospital can be taken to help alleviate the stress from hospitalization?
   a. Ensure complete separation of owners and pets
   b. Allow frequent visits and progress reports
   c. Feeding a different food so that the animal is not reminded of home
   d. Wrapping the animal tightly in warm blankets

8. What is palliative care?
   a. Advanced diagnostics when cancer is suspected
   b. Relieving of symptoms at any stage of an illness
   c. End-of-life care
   d. Euthanasia preparation

9. What is involved in developing a palliative care plan?
   a. Goals of treatment and caregiver expectations
   b. Estimates, costs, and payments
   c. List of drugs to be used and DEA protocols
   d. Concentrate on quantity over quality of life

10. What treatments are typically involved in a multi-modal approach to pain management?
    a. Surgical removal and ice packs
    b. Fluffy towels and skin care
    c. NSAIDs and opioids
    d. Yummy food and fresh water

11. What is the goal of an emergency comfort kit?
    a. To ensure the client has enough skills to treat any problem
    b. To provide clients with prescription medications in the event of a medical crisis
    c. To prevent the client from contacting the team after hours
    d. To allow the client to perform the euthanasia at home themselves

12. How is the Glasgow Feline Composite Measure Pain Scale used to identify a painful patient?
    a. Uses ear position and muzzle shape to identify pain levels
    b. Application of the probe detects increased catecholamines associated with pain
    c. Using electrical impedance, pain pathways can be determined and measured
    d. The reaction to the withdrawal of pain medications is measured

13. In what way are set points helpful in treating terminal illnesses?
    a. They establish a specific date past which care will not be continued
    b. They set a specific amount of money that will be devoted to patient care
    c. They can help determine when quality of life no longer exists for that animal
    d. They prevent the patient from starving to death

14. What would be an example of an unrealistic expectation for at-home respite care?
    a. To have one person solely responsible
    b. That medications be available for emergency use
    c. To invite neighbors and other family members in to help
    d. The hospice team continues to be involved in the care

15. What type of records need to be kept during hospice care?
    a. Medical records by the team
    b. Client assessments
    c. Medications administered and response
    d. All of the above

16. What interventions can contribute to patient comfort?
    a. Clean, soft bedding
    b. Reinforced cage with locking gate
    c. Stairs and furniture
    d. Easy to clean, slick floors

17. When is the best time to discuss euthanasia or natural death options?
    a. At the wellness examinations
    b. At the onset of hospice care
    c. After the animal has become unresponsive
    d. After death has been pronounced

18. What is a sign seen at the early stages of active dying?
    a. Loss of consciousness
    b. Cold extremities
    c. Restlessness
    d. Dark colored urine

19. What is a sign seen at the final phase of active dying?
    a. Increased sleeping
    b. Muscle spasms
    c. Confusion
    d. Inability to heal wounds

20. What role do analgesics play in active dying?
    a. They are unneeded, as the animal no longer can feel pain
    b. Due to concerns over addiction or dependence, they are unwarranted
    c. If signs of pain are noted, they can be given at the higher range of the dose
    d. Drug diversion concerns with clients restrict the use of analgesics

21. If euthanasia is performed in the clinic, how can this be made easier?
    a. Use of a quiet, secluded room
    b. Placement in the treatment room with all of the needed monitoring equipment
    c. Having the client wait in their car until just before the animal is ready to pass
    d. Heavy sedation in the kennel

22. What is an important consideration when looking to select a drug to perform a euthanasia?
    a. Clinic cost
    b. Reliability
    c. Site euthanasia is performed at
    d. Client choice

23. At the end of a successful euthanasia, what color would you expect the mucous membrane to be?
    a. Pink
    b. Bright red
    c. Blue
    d. Gray

24. Who is responsible for ensuring all laws are followed in disposing of a deceased pet?
    a. The owners
    b. The technician
    c. The veterinarian
    d. The city council

25. An animal who has been hospitalized should have what done with the catheters and monitoring devices after they have died?
    a. They remain as the owner has already paid for them
    b. The owner can decide what is removed and what remains
    c. The veterinarian in charge decides what is removed
    d. All medical paraphernalia should be removed

26. After an animal has passed, whether from natural causes or euthanasia, it is normal for clients to feel what?
    a. Relief
    b. Happiness it is over
    c. Hunger
    d. Empowered

27. When sending an animal home with the owners for burial, how is the body prepared?
    a. They are placed in the largest bag that can accommodate their body
    b. All bodies must be frozen before they can go home, so the owner will need to come back the next day to pick up the body
    c. Wrapped gently with a blanket to appear as if sleeping
    d. The animal control officer will come to pick up all bodies for disposal

28. When performing a burial of their pet at home, what should clients be informed of?
    a. Removal from any plastic wrapping is needed
    b. Blankets or towels are prohibited even in rural settings
    c. Shallow burial will result in quicker decomposition
    d. To anticipate that the groundwater will become contaminated from the drugs used, making it undrinkable

29. After a cremation, it is important for owners to know what information?
    a. That the ashes cannot be returned
    b. That ashes can be returned, but only with a private cremation
    c. That ashes are toxic and should never be handled or used for memorials
    d. That only human crematoriums can perform this service

30. What kind of anchor is provided to the client by using taxidermy or freeze-drying preservation?
    a. Visual
    b. Verbal
    c. Scent
    d. Sound

31. What options are available for the client and patient if the clinic is unable to offer hospice care?
    a. Transfer care to a veterinary hospice service
    b. To push the clinic to provide this care even when not possible
    c. To demand that the veterinarian come to their home
    d. To post on social media complaining about the clinic

32. What type of clients can be expected to show the most grief after the death of their pet?
    a. New clients who have just spent a lot of money
    b. Owners who have little attachment
    c. Those with a strong bond
    d. Anyone who lives with an animal

33. What information needs to be provided to clients when describing the grieving process?
    a. This is a linear path, and all steps must be followed
    b. Grieving only occurs when clients are deeply bonded
    c. All family members will grieve the same way
    d. Grief is individual and nonlinear

34. Which stage of grief is seen first?
    a. Anger
    b. Bargaining
    c. Denial
    d. Guilt

35. With anger from grief, who is this typically directed at?
    a. The veterinary team
    b. The family
    c. The pet
    d. Social media

36. Which stage is seen as the core of the grieving process?
    a. Denial
    b. Bargaining
    c. Sorrow
    d. Resolution

37. When clients have reached this stage, they can usually consider adoption of a new pet.
    a. Denial
    b. Bargaining
    c. Sorrow
    d. Resolution

38. When a client presents with a new pet that they have neglected, this usually indicates what?
    a. Lack of bonding
    b. Anger
    c. Bargaining
    d. Continued sorrow

39. How can we address grieving with our clients without being professional counselors?
    a. Being emotionally supportive
    b. Meeting anger with scientific facts
    c. Ensuring that only clients with active accounts will be seen
    d. Offering them a new pet at every conversation

40. One skill that can be effective when working with grieving clients is what kind of listening?
    a. Absent
    b. Distant
    c. Reflective
    d. Letting them know you know exactly how they feel

41. What is an example of open body language that encourages communication?
    a. Standing across the examination table from the client
    b. Leaning against the counter with your arms and legs crossed
    c. Looking at your notes while talking with the client
    d. Sitting next to them with your arms and legs uncrossed

42. Effective listening may involve periods of what?
    a. Silence
    b. Yelling
    c. Anger
    d. Listing of problems

43. Validating client feelings of loss can provide what to clients?
    a. A target for their anger
    b. Make them feel special and cared for
    c. Making them more despondent
    d. A means of denial

44. When performing an in-office euthanasia, when should the fees be collected?
    a. As soon as the client arrives at the front desk
    b. After the paperwork is signed, but before they enter the comfort room
    c. In the comfort room, before the euthanasia is performed
    d. After the euthanasia, at the front desk

45. How can grief associated with patient loss be dealt with by the veterinary team?
    a. Just move on quickly to the next patient
    b. Empathize and assist with team members
    c. Designate one person to be responsible for all cases that day
    d. Decide to not discuss the losses

46. What role can a positive client experience have on the hospital?
    a. Positive referrals to friends
    b. High client turnover
    c. Negative social media posts driving business
    d. Ensure only new puppy and kitten examinations are seen

47. What role can a compounded loss have on a client?
    a. None, each loss is treated individually
    b. If they are different breeds, there is no significance
    c. Each loss can build on unresolved loss from others
    d. This only pertains to losses within the immediate 6–12 months

48. If the veterinary team is concerned over a client's safety after a loss, what options are available?
    a. Referral to appropriate professionals
    b. Sweep them under the rug as they are not veterinary related
    c. Notify the police immediately
    d. Avoid all contact with the client

49. When compiling a list of referral and support services for grieving clients, where is a good place to start?
    a. The animal control officer for your county
    b. The local mental health department
    c. The state hospital

50. What sort of options can we offer to a client that is lonely but is unable to establish a new bond?
    a. Fostering
    b. Quiet time alone
    c. Retail therapy
    d. Road trip

CASE SCENARIO

Sparky is a 12-year-old F/s Labrador Retriever who has had a chronic history of hip dysplasia and has recently developed multicentric lymphoma. Her owners have been treating her with multimodal pain management for hip pain, but she has become increasingly immobile. With the development of the lymphoma, she is unable to get up by herself, and the owners have been carrying her outside and supporting her to use the bathroom.

Sparky's increasing immobility has been challenging for the owners, and they have made an appointment today to discuss what options are available for continued care with her.

You want to introduce the Colorado Pain Scale for Dogs to Sparky's family so that the veterinary team can ensure that her pain is being managed appropriately. To review the Colorado Pain Scale, go to https://vetmedbiosci.colostate.edu/vth/wp-content/uploads/sites/7/2020/12/canine-pain-scale.pdf.

After going through this pain scale the team can see that her discomfort is at a 3.5. Her owners have decided to not pursue treatment for her lymphoma.

In discussion with Dr. Smith the decision is made to enter Sparky into your palliative care program, to ensure her continued comfort. With palliative care treatment, what is the overall goal?

_____

_____

Dr. Smith will be adding opioids to her treatment plan, as well as a warming bed. The decision was made by her owners to only offer food and water if she was interested and not force the issue. Within 3 days Sparky is refusing all food and water, but her pain scale assessment is a 2. Dr. Smith recommends a transition to hospice care at this time. How do palliative care and hospice care differ?

_____

_____

As Sparky enters hospice care at home, a member of the veterinary team visits them daily and reviews her treatment plan as well as addresses her owner's concerns in communication with Dr. Smith. Two end points are set by her owners to guide the team toward the final decision to euthanize her.

Their end points are as follows: they are unable to control her pain at home and she is unwilling to engage with the family.

You want to cover options for after Sparky has passed, what options can you provide her owners?

_____

_____

Three days after entering hospice care, the owners can see that Sparky is ready. Your clinic offers both in-home euthanasia and in-clinic ones. The owners elect an at-home euthanasia and request one for the end of the day. This is set up with the receptionist, and Dr. Smith is notified. When does the payment get collected as well as information on taking care of the body?

_____

_____

Sparky's euthanasia goes smoothly, and her body is picked up by the local animal cremation service. The owners picked out a lovely urn last week but are interested in other memorial options that might be available to them. What information can you provide them on these types of services?

_____

_____

The veterinary team contacted Sparky's owners a week after she had passed to see how they were doing. Mrs. Johnson is having some challenges, as she works from home and she and Sparky have been constant office companions for the last couple of years. What support options can you provide for her?

_____

_____

Four months after Sparky's passing, her owners have adopted a 2-year-old foster from the local shelter. She has been named Iris and is nicely filling the empty hole in their lives. They understand that Iris will never replace Sparky, but they enjoy the young dog's exuberance and the changes this has offered in their lives.